The Facial Hair Handbook

Praise for
The Facial Hair Handbook

"The guy's got swagger in spades...and that attitude comes through on the pages. That makes the book a fun read – even if your aspirations for facial adornment never move beyond the milk-mustache phase."

Adam Tschorn, LA Times

"Nobody knows more about beards than Jack Passion. And if there is someone out there who knows almost as much, there's no question that Passion is more eloquent, driven and bad-ass... Behind that shock of red hair is a philosopher, a mystic, a man who very well already knows the meaning of life."

Matt Villano, SF Chronicle

"I recommend every man have two things: A beard and this book."

Phil Olsen, Captain of Beard Team USA

THE
FACIAL HAIR
HANDBOOK

Every Man's Guide To Growing
& Grooming Great Facial Hair

Jack Passion

San Francisco - Los Angeles - New York - London

Special Thanks: Mom, James Milton and the Fryes, Phil Olsen, Chris Boyd, and Alexis Klein.

The Facial Hair Handbook
Copyright © 2009 by Jack Passion

Published by Jack Passion, LLC.
jackpassion.com
facialhairhandbook.com

Library of Congress Control Number: 2009904283

ISBN: 978-0-615-29159-8

Photography by Chris Boyd.

Revised Second Printing.

Table of Contents

Foreword
By Phil Olsen
Captain - Beard Team USA

Jack Passion is to the sport of bearding what Tiger Woods is to the sport of golf.

At the tender age of 21, an age when many men still can't yet grow a decent beard, Jack burst onto the international bearding scene at the World Beard and Moustache Championships in Berlin, Germany. There he podiumed against a field made up mostly of beards older than Jack himself, putting the beardsmen who had invented the sport and thought they owned it on notice that the game itself had changed. Two years later at the next championships in Brighton, England, Jack stole the show as he walked away with top honors in the most competitive category, full beard natural, earning himself the right to claim the title "World Beard Champion." At the 2009 worlds in Anchorage, Alaska, Jack repeated his feat, taking top honors in his category once again.

In *The Facial Hair Handbook* Jack Passion examines all facets of bearding, with the same panache, confidence, and yes, passion, with which Tiger approaches an eagle putt on 18. Read this book and you will soon be on your way to rocking a great beard yourself.

Nobody does beards better.

Phil Olsen
Captain, Beard Team USA

Preface

Since the dawn of humankind, men have grown facial hair. Political leaders, religious icons, heroes, villains... Every man had a hairy face, because that's what men were supposed to look like. However, the early 1900's saw the birth of the disposable razor and a male beauty market was born. Soon, shaving became a practice for 90% of men in the world! By telling men that they weren't clean or hygienic, companies could continue to sell them razors and shaving cream. Today, men's shaving is a multi-billion dollar industry!

It should have been seen as a sign that a man can shave every day of his life and his beard will keep growing back. Over the past few years, we've seen facial hair sprouting up everywhere. Hollywood actors, musicians, and hipsters have all started wearing facial hair again. However, these groups traditionally stay abreast of the trends. Facial hair's comeback has been too slow and steady to only be a trend. It has gone beyond irony, mustache parties, and beard competitions.

We're now seeing mainstream men everywhere with facial hair. Even accountants, lawyers, doctors, and politicians have begun experimenting with facial hair. But it's not always just as easy as putting the razor to rest...

Any man will surely go back to shaving when his beard starts to itch. When a goatee or mustache looks bad, he'll shave it off, discouraged and unaware of his options. Marginalized facial hair stereotypes prevent every day, normal guys from making facial hair part of their personal style. Sadly, men have forgotten what to do with their beards and how to care for them. Until now.

The Facial Hair Handbook is the definitive guide to all aspects of facial hair. From making the decision to wear facial hair, to the best way to take it off, all men can finally be stylish and care for their appearance while staying true to who they are: Men.

Who Should Read This Book

This book is for the man who is ready to look like one.

It does not matter your race, ethnicity, sexual orientation, or age. All that matters is your sex: If you are a man, this book is for you.

The Facial Hair Handbook is not about the history of facial hair, nor is it about its place in cultures of the world. It is not the manifesto of a movement to bring facial hair back to mainstream acceptance.

Consider this book a both style guide and a motivational treatise, for men who want their personal style to include wearing facial hair. With its help, you will achieve the best, most beautiful facial hair your DNA will permit, and be able to style it to perfection. You will know what you're doing and why you're doing it.

Men unwilling to care for themselves and their appearance can put this book down and go back to a life of shorn shame. Care and maintenance for your face and grooming the hair that grows on it often takes much more time than shaving would.

Too long has facial hair been marginalized by a small handful of stereotypes. Mainstream men of all ages are growing facial hair and this is their guide to doing it with style.

How to Read
The Facial Hair Handbook

The Facial Hair Handbook is divided into two sections.

- Part I is the theory of facial hair; the philosophy; a motivational treatise.

- Part II is the practice; practical advice for grooming; easy-to-follow steps.

The book can be used as a reference, but it follows the lifecycle of facial hair from growing, to grooming, to getting rid. The most effective usage would be to read the book completely, and then keep it close at hand for quick advice.

Don't forget to check out the website at facialhairhandbook.com for updated tips, product reviews, and news about facial hairstyle and care.

Disclaimer

I have a huge beard. You don't need to want or have a huge beard to read and benefit from this book. While I will address the needs of those with really long and/or thick beards, *The Facial Hair Handbook* is written for **every** man, and **every** facial hairstyle. Personally, I feel it is more impressive to see a short, well-groomed beard than a long unruly one, but Big Red has become part of my personal style, so I abide.

Whatever your preferred style, it is essential that your facial hair be maintained, *especially* if you choose to grow a big long one. This book will guide you in that maintenance.

I would also like to add that I am not a doctor or a scientist. I do, however, have one of the greatest beards in *history*. As such, this book is the result of experience and research. I have made every effort to provide the most pertinent, useful information – information that has proven effective for myself and thousands of others – in the most simple and succinct format possible. However, just as facial hair varies from man to man, so might your results.

Part I:
Growing

Getting Ready

The decision to grow and wear facial hair is not one to be taken lightly. This chapter focuses on what you need to know *before* you start growing it out.

To Be(ard)

There are many reasons to grow facial hair. If you're reading this book, chances are you've already made the decision to take the fate of your face into your own hands. To begin, I'd like to discuss some of the philosophical reasons for growing a beard.

Facial Hair Makes You a Man

Facial hair is a secondary sex characteristic that begins growing during puberty on most male humans. Women will sometimes grow facial hair, but that discussion is outside the scope of this book. Facial hair growth accelerates during adolescence, when male sex hormones start to kick into high gear. Pubic hair, broader shoulders, and a deeper voice all accompany facial hair during your passage into manhood. Facial hair makes you a man.

To put it into perspective, consider a couple of the secondary sex characteristics of the human female that signify her maturity into womanhood: The growth of breasts and the widening of hips. Looks (and feels) like signs of a good mate, wouldn't you agree? Likewise, on a primal, instinctual level, facial hair is a sign that you are a healthy and virile male.

Speaking purely biologically, with no consideration of culture and social construction of masculinity and femininity, the dichotomy of the sexes is what makes them attracted to one another. We don't grow breasts; women don't grow facial hair. Celebrate what makes you a man.

One of the stumbling blocks of the metrosexual movement was that it didn't account for men who wanted to maintain a traditionally masculine image while paying close attention to their appearance. Facial hair is the perfect avenue for stylish, masculine expression. You can get your nails done, and then walk across the street and get your beard done!

Facial Hair is the Human Plumage

In birds, the male of the species carries the plumage. Just look at them: Female birds usually have subdued, darker colors, to help guard and camouflage them. The males, on the other hand, have all the bright colors and markings to compete for and attract the females. The most famous example of this is obviously the peacock. Examples of sexual dimorphism can be seen elsewhere in the animal kingdom, too. For instance, the male lion wears his plumage in the form of a mane. Maybe you should too.

Facial Hair is Unique to Its Face

All men grow very different facial hair. Return, for a moment, to the animal metaphor, and think of facial hair differences as our markings. The hair grows in different patterns, different colors (often different from our head hair), begins higher or lower on the face or neck, has patches in certain places, etc. And this is even before it's styled! If you saw three men, one with a grey beard, one with a black mustache, and one with a pencil red mustache, you'd easily remember which one was which. Just as much as a jaw line or eye color makes our faces different, so does our facial hair.

Once upon a time, men wore beards to be all they could be in battle. Now we shave our soldiers and cut their hair all the same to strip them of their individuality; an army of one. What kind of warrior are you?

Facial Hair Is Personal Style

Clothes don't make the man. But clothes can make the man feel good, can make his first impression a lasting one, and can define his style. If you haven't figured it out yet, I like to bring things back to a primitive, human nature level. I feel like a lot of issues in our culture today (the abandonment of wearing facial hair notwithstanding) come about because we've perhaps forgotten who we are a little bit. We are many things, but humans are undeniably visual animals. Evolution of our media influenced culture has only made us *more* visually mindful. You may have the best personality and fit every possible definition of success, but people are still going to look at you.

I'm not suggesting you need to look a certain way, I'm just saying you need **to be aware that you do**. Men's fashion and style are outside the scope of this book. There are books about men's style, but it changes so frequently, so I'd recommend checking with magazines for what is current. A variety of factors – social, cultural, economic, and personal – will dictate what you wear and how you present yourself to the world.

Personal style transcends fashion. Even the most fringe chichi fashion designers all respect and aim for one thing: Personal style. What you wear is important, but *how* you wear it is more important. This goes for clothing as well as facial hair. Good facial hair will enhance your image above and beyond your fashion sense.

We know your facial hair is unique to you, so consider it an accessory that nobody else can have or wear. **Limited edition? Try one of a kind.** And that's what personal style is about: Setting yourself apart from everyone else and doing it with style.

Facial Hair Commands Respect

Facial hair has always been a sign of virility, wisdom, experience, and masculinity. It takes time to cultivate good facial hair, and its wearer has endured the passage of that time. He has grown into manhood. He is a healthy sexual animal. He decides his appearance for himself.

Most men would prefer to wear facial hair, but they don't because of work or women. When they see you wearing facial hair, other men will immediately respect you for having the balls to be your own man.

On the other hand, bad facial hair commands zero respect. In fact, it makes you look bad, and it makes us all look bad. Know when to say when and keep it groomed. We'll get to this later in the book.

Facial Hair is Cool

Facial hair works like a scar or a tattoo as a "cool" accessory. I know I'm playing into some of the age-old facial hair stereotypes that this book seeks to dissolve, but facial hair definitely makes you a badass. Bikers, mountain men, loggers, truckers, Jack Passion, Chuck Norris, Alaskan fishermen, Vikings, pirates, Magnum PI... These are legendary men of Awesome, and they all rock facial hair. Kicking ass and growing facial hair go together. You can chew bubble gum, too, but be careful with the bubbles.

Facial Hair is Iconic

Maybe it's just its ability to set you apart from other men, but facial hair can transform you into a legend. So many famous faces are made instantly recognizable by their facial hair. Iconic facial hair includes that of Jesus Christ, Einstein, Hitler, Elvis Presley, and ZZ Top. Heroes or villains, if you're a man worth remembering, you're a man with facial hair.

Now imagine what facial hair can do for *your* image. Even if you don't normally wear facial hair, a simple beard can really help out. Search on the Internet for "George Clooney Beard," and see how much attention is given to the man when he wears a beard.

Furthermore, facial hair is a great conversation starter, for business or pleasure. I've gotten many jobs just simply because I stood out and could break the ice and set a good tone talking about my beard. Girls talk to me first (usually about my beard), so I don't even have to try. If you work with people, in sales, real estate, or in entertainment, try distinct facial hair to set you apart from your competitors.

If your face is your brand, use it!

Facial Hair is Commitment

It takes a good amount of time to cultivate good facial hair. And as you will find, its rewards do not come without some sacrifice. Your beard will itch, you will have bad (facial) hair days, and women will laugh (Just be glad they're laughing at your face!). But if you can hold out, you're going to love what you've done. You are going to feel really accomplished, and proud of yourself. I promise you: You're going to love it. And people are going to respect you for putting in the time to do something cool.

Facial hair growth contests are often held to show support for a good cause. Some only last a month: Manuary, Mustache March, and Novembeard, for instance. Others go until someone shaves: Whoever shaves first loses (obviously).

The NHL playoff beard is a commitment to your team as they play their way to the Stanley Cup. When your team loses, you have to shave. Moral of the story? **Losers shave**.

They say that Rome wasn't built in a day, but that Disneyland was built in a year and a day. Disneyland's the happiest place on Earth! Put in some time and yours can be the happiest *face* on Earth!

Facial Hair is Meaningful

Facial hair is often associated with religion, culture, or ceremony. *Every* major religion of the world mentions guidelines for wearing facial hair in its accompanying text. Most of the time, it turns out that the Word is in favor of facial hair.

Ask any man with facial hair about it and he will undoubtedly have a story. Facial hair can carry many meanings, even if only to its wearer.

Facial Hair is Temporary

Facial hair *isn't* a tattoo. It's *not* a scar. And it's *not* plastic surgery. But it still carries the weight of meaningful expression and experience. It still allows you to shape and change your face, while being natural and authentically masculine.

You can try different styles very easily. If you mess up, you can always shave and start again. The hair will always grow back! All the while, you look like the man.

Facial Hair Protects Your Skin

Protection is one of the biological reasons our faces grow hair in the first place. When your skin has hair on it, it won't get wrinkles. You never need to exfoliate under your facial hair. It's great at protecting from the elements, as well.

Sun and wind just can't get to your skin to damage it, and your beard keeps you warm in cold weather. The first thing men always tell me when they shave off a beard is how cold it is without the beard. Men from Northern ancestry typically have more facial hair as well. Like a dog built for the snow, so are we for the cold. Try a full beard in the winter months to keep your face protected in outdoor conditions. One of the most insightful sights is when you see a skier's beard covered in ice. All that cold icy air got caught in the beard instead of freezing the face!

No discussion of the cold can be complete without the cold *hearted*. If you get yourself in trouble and a woman tries to slap you, a beard will absorb the impact of a facial slap. It just won't hurt! And she'll probably change her mind as soon as she feels that manly beard anyway!

There Are Many Other Reasons To Grow and Wear Facial Hair:

To look older
To look younger
To look like Jack Passion (You'd better hit the gym, too…)
To rebel
To avoid shaving
To shape your face
To make up for balding
To hide a double chin
To hide a blemish
To hide stuff
To hide out
Etc.

The Best Reason to Grow Facial Hair

Every man I talk to is proud of his facial hair. It makes you a man, but it makes you your own man. It's cool, but it's your own brand of cool. I often ask men, "How can you know who you are if you don't know what you're supposed to look like?" In the journey of self-discovery, you can learn a lot about yourself by just not shaving for a little while.

There's an element of spirituality involved as well. You are embracing yourself and the body you inhabit, and maintaining your facial hair can be as meditative as prayer. Does God want you to have a beard? Guys tell me all the time that they'd never even considered that they could grow a beard, and how excited they are at the thought of doing it. I ask them why, and they can't explain it.

That's because the best reason to grow facial hair cannot be explained; only experienced. Growing a beard or a mustache can be a serious, life-changing event. It's also a lot of fun. Whatever your reason, this is definitely one of those times to enjoy the journey.

Not to Be(ard)

Despite the aforementioned truths, which I hold to be self-evident, there are a few reasons you shouldn't wear facial hair.

Sometimes, You Just Look Better Without Facial Hair

There are many reasons for this: Maybe it's patchy, maybe it's asymmetrical, or maybe it makes you look like the local sex offender. The chapter *Getting Good* addresses what can be done to grow a better beard, but know that you can wear stubble in the meantime, and that your ability to grow facial hair will get better as you get older.

Sometimes, You Need to Get Paid

There are some professions that require you to keep your face shorn. If you've tried keeping your beard groomed or only wearing a mustache, and the boss still threatens to let you go, think about shaving before thinking about another job. I discuss the vacation beard in the chapter *Getting Started*, so even if you can't look awesome every day, just know that you have one more thing to look forward to when you're not working!

Sometimes, You Need to Get Laid

Perhaps you are involved in a romantic relationship with a woman who just does not want you to have facial hair. Brother, I hope she's smoking hot and has a lot of money, because she obviously doesn't care about you and what you want. Her friends probably suck, she probably listens to horrible music, and she probably can't cook. Your sex life is probably passionless, and she's probably a real bitch. My advice? Embezzle her money, put up with her bullshit as long as you can, then hire me to seduce her. Use her infidelity to get rid of her, and then live off the cash you stashed. Know this: I'll always take one for the bearded team, and I'm good at the bitchy ones. Also, I only assume heterosexuality here because gay men usually embrace the beard, making this one a non-issue for them.

Sometimes, It Can Go Either Way

Look at Sean Connery. The man was a sex symbol playing James Bond with a clean-shaven face, and now he's a legend who wears his beard no matter what role he's cast in. Brad Pitt, while famous for his looks sans-beard, wore a substantial beard for a while, kept it well groomed, and looked fantastic wherever he went. As of this writing, he's wearing a goatee. Note though, that in both men's cases, their looks were made *even more* distinctive with facial hair; both kept themselves and their images fresh and updated by continually reinventing themselves with facial hair.

The important thing to note here though is that while you might look better without facial hair, there's only one way to find out. Grow it out and experiment. If it's just not happening, it should be completely obvious.

Why It Grows

Facial hair is a secondary sex characteristic of human males that begins to grow during puberty and is the result of a number of factors including genetics, hormones, and health. We've covered a lot of philosophical reasons you should grow facial hair, but now let's discuss the biological reasons it grows in the first place.

One explanation is for protection. Hair protects skin. People whose ancestry comes from harsh climates will often have hair traits that match the conditions of those climates. Big thick beards protect the face from the cold and the wind just like big, bushy eyebrows protect the eyes from desert sand. Pubic hair supposedly protects the genitals (in my opinion, you're better off using a condom). Is this relevant in today's world? Absolutely not! Evolution has left men with hair in certain places on our body, just as it's left us with nipples. But since neither facial hair, nor nipples have proven any evolutionary threat, they haven't been evolutionarily disposed of, either.

That said, hair does still protect the body, and your facial hair will help keep your face looking young and healthy. We'll discuss this more later, but along the same lines, I believe the only relevant remaining biological reason we grow facial hair is to display our overall health.

Humans are here to do three things: eat, sleep, and procreate. Life is usually, or at least should usually, be about sustaining these activities. Everything else is a distraction and a complication. The "Meaning of Life" has always been to survive, just as it is for any other living thing on the planet. Only in recent times has survival become guaranteed enough to even consider there might be any other reason to live.

We know that humans are visual animals, and visual attraction is definitely part of our mating ritual. For example, men in the modern meat market we call dating will look at a woman and think, "Good body, good to go," and they've got enough information to select their mate. Women look at men, too, but the process is a bit more complex. They infer things about us from what they learn visually. When a woman sees a man driving a nice car, she isn't attracted to the nice car: She's attracted to what got him that car. She infers that he must have the money to get that kind of car, and if he's got that kind of money to support himself, he can probably support her and their offspring, too. Obviously, dating and mating is *far* more complicated than this, but we can't ignore the fact that men and women are checking each other out.

Now let's go back to better times when we were all roaming this planet naked, and we didn't have to have nice cars to get chicks. Women had to use more natural methods to select a healthy, virile mate from the crowd. Fortunately, the human body displays its own sign of successful distinction: Hair.

The body has many functions, but things like good hair, skin, and nails *only* occur when the body is functioning optimally. In the primal, visceral, sexual corners of her mind, good hair lets a woman know you are capable of providing the nutrients to grow that good hair, and make the shelter to keep it nice. **Hair indicates health**. To grow good hair, including facial hair, you need to be healthy. **It's that simple**.

Facial hair, specifically, is the result of testosterone. Testosterone, we know, is the male sex hormone. When you have healthy facial hair, it can only be because you are healthy, physically *and* sexually. Therefore, your facial hair identifies you has a healthy mate.

Thus, we arrive at the following.

> ## Passion's 1st Law of Facial Hair
> Healthy Man, Healthy Beard

It's amazing what the human body can go through. Your body can survive through malnutrition and illness like a champ – from something as simple as being dehydrated with chapped lips, to shriveling up after months without food. Apropos to our discussion: If you're hormonally weak and malnourished, you're just not going to be the prime pick for pumping!

Your facial hair, in good condition, shows you're in good condition. This is how the beard became a sign of virility. This is why fierce warriors were intimidating with beards. This is why I win beard competitions. The same steps that take you to healthy facial hair or skin are the same steps that take you to overall health. And vice versa, if you want to grow a good beard, you need to grow a good man. It's win-win: Health is wealth, nice car or no nice car.

Why It Doesn't Grow

If you don't have any facial hair, don't worry. Here are a couple of things to consider:

Facial Hair may begin growing during puberty, but it often doesn't accelerate until later. You might not start growing thick hair until your thirties or forties, and that's perfectly normal. We're all different.

Some men grow less facial hair than others. You just might not be a hairy guy, and that's not a problem. It may limit what you can do style-wise, but it doesn't mean you're any less of a man, or that you can't wear what facial hair you do have. Stereotypes that certain races cannot grow facial hair are unfounded. Again, facial hair can really start growing later in their life. Most, but definitely not all, people inherit their hair from their mom's dad. Look at your maternal grandfather for a good idea of what you can expect and when you can expect it.

If you suspect a hormone imbalance or something else serious, see a doctor. There will usually be other signs to indicate something isn't working right, but since testosterone and facial hair are linked, it cannot be ruled out. Excessive facial hair growth in women is usually the result of and one of the first signs of hormone imbalance.

If you are in poor health, you will not grow facial hair. The body turns certain functions off so it can continue to survive with the essentials. Stress, poor diet, liver condition, poor sleep patterns, serious illness, drug abuse, and even mild, functioning dehydration can all stop your facial hair from growing.

Life in the Pash Lane

One time, I got food poisoning from some bad chicken. I won't go into details, but I lost 15 lbs that night, and another 15 in the weeks that followed. I was really sick, and recovery took almost a month. That month ruined my beard. Hairs fell out of my face left and right, and growth unquestionably halted. I still won't eat chicken to this day unless I buy and cook it myself.

Remember the first law of facial hair: Healthy Man, Healthy Beard. If you're living a healthy lifestyle, you will grow facial hair to the best of your ability. It's not about the most; it's about the best.

Key Points

- There are a lot of reasons to grow facial hair and only a few reasons not to.

- Facial hair is an important part of being a man.

- Facial hair can help you achieve personal style.

- You might look better without facial hair, but the only way you're going to know that is if you see what it looks like on you first.

- You might look good with *and* without facial hair. Change it up! "Variety is the spice of life."

- Passion's 1st Law of Facial Hair: Healthy Man, Healthy Beard.

- Hair condition shows health condition, and facial hair evolved to show your sexual health condition.

Getting Started

Whatever style you decide to wear, you have to get some hair on your face first. This chapter discusses describes how to begin growing a beard.

Start with a Beard

Passion's 2nd Law of Facial Hair
Good Facial Hair Starts With a Beard

You've got to grow out the crop before you can harvest it. There are several reasons for this:

First, the growth of the beard covers enough of the face that it can sneak on without drawing too much attention to itself. If you try to bring a mustache out on its own, for instance, it's going to take several weeks. All the while, you are going to look like the sleaziest mullet-rocking, El Camino-driving, drug dealer that's ever lived. If you're going to do this, you've got to do it with style, and beard stubble is a style itself.

Second, it's hard (and by hard I mean impossible) to know what's going to look best until you see what you're working with. When you're growing a mustache or a goatee, you can't trim or shave symmetrically from the start. You need to grow out a beard, *and then* shave off what you don't want. The same goes for sideburns. As we'll see, it's easy to draw shaving guidelines in your beard with a comb. (Sure, you could use a pen, but then you'd be ugly *and* have pen all over your face).

If you've never grown out your beard before, you might not know how your hair grows. There might be blank patches or curls, and we're going to need to figure out the grain of your hair. It's essential to know what you've got before you can style it into something. You might think you're going to have a mustache, and upon growing out the beard, decide you want to have a soul patch with that 'stache. Or you might have a weak mustache, but an otherwise great beard with which to compensate.

Men who have had different facial hairstyles will agree: Start with a beard.

Life in the Posh Lane
I never knew that I was going to grow a beard. I started the beard I have today with the intention of cutting it into another style. It turned out to be such an awesome beard, though, that I kept it a beard.

Baby Beard
To *start* growing a beard, you need to *stop* shaving. This is very easy. In fact, the first few weeks of growing a beard is how beards get their reputation for laziness. Just let it go.

Depending on how fast you grow facial hair, you might want to time this effectively. Beasts blessed with black five o'clock shadow at ten in the morning are good to go. You'll have a beard in a day or two, and in the meantime, you'll be wearing stubble, which is a perfectly acceptable facial hairstyle. In fact, it's the favorite of most women.

The color of your facial hair also factors into this decision. Blonde and red beards are going to need at least a week before they start to look like stubble. Guys with patchy or not so thick facial hair will need some time to get it long enough to cover up the holes. The beginning stages can look awful. You will potentially look sick and dirty, so make sure to maintain the rest of your appearance!

Try this schedule to jump-start your beard without letting people see the weak stage:

Thursday Don't shave. Go to work as normal. People will just think you didn't shave that day. Not a problem.

Friday If you started Thursday, call in sick and stay home. Sleep most of the day, eat steak, and drink plenty of water. Read the rest of this book.

Saturday Relax.

Sunday Relax some more.

Monday Walk past the receptionist at work with some sexy stubble, or show your boss who's boss with a burly beard. Go to your desk and write to Jack Passion and tell him his book changed your life. When the day is done, bring the receptionist home with you.

You can also begin with a Vacation Beard. The vacation beard is usually terminated at the end of the vacation, but is another great way to get a start. Get a jump-start on your vacation by starting your vacation beard on Thursday, as well.

Growing a vacation beard has two steps:
1. Go on vacation.
2. Don't shave on vacation.

If this is your first time letting your beard go, you're in for an amazing, transformational experience. Give it a little time to come in before showing people. Don't let them see the weak beginnings and make up their mind that you don't look good with facial hair before they've seen what you can do.

Stay away from people who discourage the project. Instead, find a bearded friend, or get a friend to stop shaving with you. It'll make it much easier to have someone who can relate. It takes balls to grow a beard when the world around you doesn't approve. Four balls are better than two. An army of balls is even better.

If you're following this book in sequence, I'm now going to assume you've begun growing a beard. While we've got some time, let's look at what makes a beard grow well.

Hair is Dead! Long Live the Face!

This may be the single most important paragraph in this book, so listen closely: Hair is dead. The life and growth of your facial hair happens in your face, under your skin, at the base of your hair follicle. There is nothing you can do to make your dead hair better once it's grown out. Additionally, once you've grown it out, you've got a lot of things working against it. We'll talk about how to care for the hair once it's grown, but it's essential that you grow it out right the first time so we're working with the best hair we can.

Fast Faced

There is nothing you can put on your face or your beard to make it grow faster naturally. This goes for shampoos, conditioners, oils, etc. You can use Minoxidil (Usually sold under the brand name Rogaine®) on your face, and studies have shown it will help you grow hair there, but that's cheating. Additionally, the kind of illegal steroids and human growth hormones that athletes take will definitely help you produce more testosterone and grow more facial hair. This is illegal, and it's also cheating. Plus, in both cases, there can be serious negative side effects.

Hair growth has a maximum speed, and it's different for everyone, especially with facial hair. Head hair usually grows half an inch per month, but men's faces are not only different than their scalps, but they evolve with time.

Passion's 3rd Law of Facial Hair
Hair Growth is About Potential

If you're doing everything right, you will grow good hair as fast as your body will let you, and there's nothing you can do beyond that. **All you can do is realize *your* potential**.

Contrary to popular belief, shaving your beard *will not* make it grow back thicker. Hair growth starts with a point, and gets thicker as it gets longer. The illusion of thicker hair after shaving is caused by the fact that when you shave a beard, you're cutting the hair right at the thick part of the hair, leaving yourself growing hair from a thick, flat edge.

Key Points

- Passion's 2nd Law: Good Facial Hair Starts With a Beard.

- Hair is dead. The life and growth of your facial hair happens in your face. There is nothing you can do to make your dead hair better once it's grown out.

- Passion's 3rd Law: Hair Growth is About Potential.

- If you're doing everything right, you will grow good hair as fast as your body will let you, and there's nothing you can do beyond that.

Getting Good

Diet: It Eats More Than Your Crumbs

You are what you eat, and so is your beard. A strand of hair is like a timeline of your health. Scientists use hair to examine a person's diet over a period of time. If you only get one thing from this book, let it be Passion's First Law of Facial Hair. Your beard will grow to its fullest potential when you're eating a healthy, balanced diet. There are many ways to do this, but here's some food for thought as they relate to hair: (All puns intended).

Carbohydrates

Don't buy into the low-carb hype: You need carbohydrates to live. Carbohydrates give you and your body the energy it needs to grow a beard! That said, definitely try to aim for complex carbohydrates. Some examples include fruit, vegetables, oats, whole-wheat products, pasta, oats, or beans. One of the best things you can do for yourself when selecting which carbs to eat is to look at how much fiber they have. It depends on your dietary needs, but generally speaking, the more complex the carb, the more fiber it will have, and the better it is for you. You'll get the benefits of lasting energy, a low hit to your blood sugar (You'll store less fat), and your digestion will be much easier. High-fiber food is good beard food because it's good man food. There is lots of evidence that supports a diet high in fiber can prevent heart disease and colon cancer, two very serious concerns for men. I'm not going to lie though; the satisfaction of a high fiber diet is found in the bathroom.

Avoid sugar. Sugar is addictive and will make you sick, fat, ugly, and unhappy. Furthermore, it is well known that sugar grows brittle, easily breakable hair. Limiting your intake of processed sugar is one of the healthiest things you can do for yourself, bearded or not bearded, but especially bearded.

Protein
Hair is essentially protein, so it's a very important part of your diet for maximum beard potential. Protein rich foods include meat, poultry, fish, dairy products, nuts, and legumes. There are countless benefits to a vegetarian diet, but for efficient maximization of protein intake, animal sources will always have more protein. Additionally, animal protein sources have important B vitamins and minerals essential to good hair growth.

However, there are health risks with eating red meat, and almost all fish contains deadly contaminants. There is a lot of evidence against dairy, as well. Whether or not you wish to eat meat in your diet is up to you. There are plenty of vegetarians and vegans in perfect health. A balanced diet will mitigate most health risks and give you a good intake of protein.

Most people get enough protein in their diet, so don't worry about this too much. You do not need to supplement your protein intake with a protein shake, just make sure you're getting some *quality* protein with every meal.

Fat

Fat plays many important roles in the body. For hair, it's what makes the casing around the hair that prevents it from cracking and breaking. The trick is to eliminate "bad fats" like trans and saturated fats; and eat "good," unsaturated fats. You have to be careful, as saturated fat is found in protein-rich and good-for-the-beard animal products (For example: eggs, steak, and seafood... damn it!); moderation is the key (in fact, your body actually benefits *some* saturated fats). Trans fats occur when oil is hydrogenated. Avoid hydrogenated anything and you should be good.

You may have heard about Omega 3 fatty acids. Found in fish, avocado, flaxseed, olive oil, and a bunch of other foods, Omega 3s are the best fat for your body. And, surprise, surprise, they're the best fat for your hair, too! Omega 3s are *essential* to hair growth, strength, and condition. Most diets do not include enough Omega 3s. Eat fish and cook with olive oil, sprinkle flax seeds on your cereal, or go California-style and put avocado on everything.

Calories

A lot of people equate "Eating healthy" with losing weight. Ideally, eating healthy will get you to your natural weight – what's healthy for *your* body. It's true that most people have a little to lose. A caloric deficit occurs when you burn more calories in a day than you take in from food, and slight deficit is a healthy way to lose weight. Be careful with weight loss, though. Rapid weight loss will impede hair growth and even cause it to fall out. And in our case, we're trying to *grow* a beard. A lot of guys with great beards are big, husky guys. Though they may be going overboard a little, they're also getting enough of what it takes to ensure their beard has enough to grow on, so I would avoid a caloric deficit for the purposes of growing a beard.

We're growing a flower on our face: We need nutrients.

And just like growing a flower, we also need water...

Water

If eliminating processed sugar isn't the best thing you can do for your health, drinking more water is. Our body is mostly water, and drinking plenty of water keeps us filtered and fresh. Tragically, most people are under-hydrated. Literally every process in our bodies uses water, including and especially hair growth. If there should exist some magical elixir that grows facial hair as fast as possible, it's water. Skimp everywhere else before you skimp on how much water you're drinking.

To reiterate: We can't make the hair any better once it's grown out. Hydration is probably the most important part of ensuring we grow the best hair out that we can. Some sources recommend drinking two liters of water a day. Consider the size of a two-liter bottle, and then think if you're drinking that much.

Vitamins and Supplements

There is no magic beard-growing supplement: All you can do is realize your potential. A quality multivitamin should be all you need. Fish oil and Flaxseed oil supplements are highly recommended, too, for their Omega 3 content. There are hair vitamins, and they usually focus on hair-nourishing B-Vitamins and Biotin, as well as the minerals like zinc, magnesium, and silica. **A good multivitamin will cover all of these**. You can take a hair-specific vitamin as well, but your body can only absorb so much. When your urine turns fluorescent, know that you're getting too many vitamins. As such, you're probably also wasting your money. There is a maximum potential for hair growth you can't pass, no matter how many vitamins you take. Go to a health food store and get help selecting a good multivitamin the first time out.

People always discuss prenatal vitamins and hair growth. Prenatal vitamins contain vitamins that help with hair and nails, but they are specially formulated for women and can inhibit healthy hormonal function in men, and therefore facial hair growth. It's not the prenatal vitamins that make women grow awesome hair and nails when they're pregnant; it's the pregnancy and resulting hormonal chemistry in their bodies themselves.

A quality multivitamin and a healthy diet is really all you need. You want to eliminate stress, too, so don't make this any harder than it needs to be.

Smoking

Smoking is a bad idea for bearding. It restricts blood and oxygen flow throughout your body, including to your face. Beard hair hold on to smells, too; you *will* smell like an ashtray. Smoking has been proven to accelerate hair loss and premature graying. Smoking will not only prevent you from growing a good one, it'll probably ruin the beard you already have! You have one chance to grow your beard at maximum potential, and smoking is the anti-beard.

And besides, once you've got a good beard going, a stray ash could set your face on fire! (More on this later, too).

Alcohol

Consumption of alcohol will not affect your facial hair at all. Some side effects of alcohol consumption might even help your beard grow (relaxation, better sleep, and more sex)! The key word with alcohol is moderation. Excessive drinking can tax your liver, and then you're looking at, you guessed it: bad hair that grows slow or won't grow at all. If you can handle your booze, you're good. Late stage alcoholic? Start growing your beard in rehab as a commitment to your sobriety.

Caffeine

Too much caffeine won't directly affect your hair, but it can definitely have negative side effects on your health. If anything, it's usually the means of administering that caffeine that have the negative effect on your health. Soda pop is full of processed sugar, and coffee is full of all kinds of roasted oils. Too much caffeine hits your body like a negative stressor, causing your heart to beat faster and your muscles to tense up. Not surprisingly, caffeine is proven to negatively affect sleep patterns. It has long been associated with dehydration, as well. Drinking coffee all day is not a good idea for good hair, or health in general, but a cup or two in the morning with a healthy lifestyle? Nothing to worry about, especially if you're getting good sleep and drinking plenty of water.

Dr. Passion

I am not a nutritionist or a dietician. This information is just meant to get you started and to highlight what's important for hair growth. I aim for simplicity in this book; consistency over perfection. If nutrition is something that interests you, I highly recommend further research on your own. Healthy eating should be an important interest for everyone. There are many ways to eat healthy, and I urge you to learn as much as you can. The beauty of hair is that it *is* **your health**. If you eat healthy diet, you will be healthy, and you will grow healthy facial hair. **It really is that simple**.

Stress and Rest

Have you ever noticed your facial hair seems to grow overnight? It's not just because you haven't looked at yourself all night. Your beard grows best while you're asleep. Moreover, testosterone production is at its highest in the morning after you've been in a deep sleep.

When you're sleeping, your body can dedicate its energy to repairing itself and growing new cells. New cells = new hair. Humans are here to do three things, and one of them is sleep. Getting enough sleep is crucial to good health and growing good hair. In primitive times, you could only sleep if you were safe with shelter. Only the strongest survivalists could ensure a good night's sleep, and those are the people we evolved from. You better believe they had beards, because we're still growing them!

Think about it like we're growing a flower again. During the day, the flower blooms; at night, it closes in on itself.

Regular, good quality sleep will make it easier to be healthier in other aspects of your life, also. Healthy sleep patterns assist in digestion and immunity. Getting enough sleep is also an important way to prevent stress.

Stress is a normal and healthy part of life, but too much of anything is a bad thing. Stress can have incredible effects on your overall health, as your body treats it just like trauma. When your body is stressed out, it turns biological functions off so it can focus on what's critical for survival. Facial hair growth is far from being critical, so it's one of the first things to go. Even if you maintain growth, long-term stress will ruin the quality of the hair you grow. Hell, it can ruin your *life*.

Stress affects everyone differently, and everyone reacts differently, so I can't tell you exactly what to expect and what you can do. And not to stress you out or anything, but no matter who you are, stress will make your hair (on your head or on your face) fall out or turn grey.

Get enough sleep and take care of what's stressing you. Your health and your beard will love you for it.

Exercise

Exercise relieves stress and helps you sleep better, and promotes new cell growth in the body. There are a couple benefits of exercise that directly impact facial hair growth.

Exercise gets your heart pumping and blood flowing through your body. In Chinese medicine, hair health is directly related to blood flow. Acupuncture and herbs for hair and blood are usually the same. There's a good reason for this: Blood flow is what carries all the nutrients throughout your body. All that healthy food we've been eating and all the water we've been drinking gets distributed throughout your body (and therefore to your face) **through your blood.**

Exercise will also promote hair growth because your body will be repairing itself. When your muscles break down during exercise, your body rebuilds them with new cells. Since you've been eating well, drinking plenty of water, and getting enough rest, this process is easy and your body will grow new hair at the same time. Plus, regular exercise keeps testosterone levels healthy. The best periods of beard growth I've had were when I was lifting weights and swimming. I was an optimized, healthy, muscle and beard growing testosterone machine! But don't even think for a second you have to be a gym rat. If hard training is a perfect 10, minimal, but regular, exercise is a close 8. This is one of those times when a little is *so much* better than nothing at all.

I've preached simplicity and balance for diet, and the same goes for exercise. Twenty minutes of simple exercise is all it takes. Daily exercise is easier than you think, and you'll feel great for it, too. Take a walk around the block, or just take the stairs when you have the option.

Or, better yet, find a workout partner and get my favorite exercise…

Sex

Sex is the single best way to boost testosterone levels. It is also great exercise, but it relieves stress and helps blood flow more than normal exercise can. It makes your immune system stronger, and will ensure you get good sleep. It will make you confident, and that can only get you more sex, which will get you more of the benefits of sex! (Confidence, as a side note, will also help you truly *rock* your facial hair). There are lots of things you can do to promote good health, but sex beats them all; it's the capstone to this entire chapter.

It's important to note that most of the health benefits from sex come from having sex with a partner. Unfortunately, at some point, someone made up some horrible rumor that women don't like facial hair. Don't worry, though. When you have good facial hair, it's going to work in your favor. We're going to get you looking sharp, and **your beard will get you laid**; I guarantee it.

In the throes of Passion, your hard work will pay off when your mate feels that beard and takes it to the next level. There's a reason porn stars have mustaches. Sex is a celebration of the authentic human in all of us, and the pleasure is nature's way of telling us it's good for us. There is no moderation necessary. Sex is the rain dance of facial hair. Make it rain!

Key Points

- Passion's 1st Law of Facial Hair: Healthy Man, Healthy Beard.

- I cannot stress this enough. Growing a good beard is very easy if you're taking care of yourself. Life in general is much easier if you're taking care of yourself. Hair is health.

- The quality of your beard is directly related to the quality of your life.

When Things Get Hairy

Ok, so your beard is starting to come in. This is when things begin to get complicated. If you wanted this to go smoothly, you'd have shaved your face smooth. Check out *When Things Get Hairy – Grooming* for complications that arise during the grooming or wearing of facial hair.

Itching

Itching is by far the most famous obstacle for facial hair growth. Fortunately, it is a simple problem with simple solutions.

Your face itches in the early stages of growing a beard for two main reasons:

The first reason is that your face, used to being clean-shaven, has not had to manage the oil necessary to protect your facial hair. Your face wants to protect the new hair, and so as the beard starts coming in more and more, it overcompensates, and your face gets really oily. There is an ebb and flow to this, so your face can get very dry too. All kinds of irritations can ensue. Basically, you have facial skin chaos.

The second reason is that some of these super short hairs are just starting to get long enough to curl back and scratch at your face. All of these hairs reaching back and tickling your face will drive you *crazy*. Most men end up shaving because of this.

Either way, **the itching will pass**. Here are some mitigating solutions to prevent you from giving up:

First of all, if you're following Passion's First Law of Facial Hair, you're going to eliminate at least half the itching. Healthy living will make for healthy skin, including on your face, and that will minimize a lot of the potential for irritation. This is the time to supplement your diet with fish and flaxseed oil, as Omega 3 fats really help with skin condition. Processed sugar, among other horrible atrocities, is famous for causing skin problems. Eliminate processed sugar and your itching will subside in strides. This alone may prevent the itching altogether.

Brush your beard. We'll discuss brushing more when we discuss grooming, as well as what kind of brush to use, but this is a great time to get started with a brush. When your beard is really short, the brush will basically be a tool for scratching your face. Your fingers will make your beard dirty with all kinds of foreign substances, oils, and bacteria, so scratching your face with your fingers will just going to make it itch more. Plus, the difference between scratching with a brush vs. your fingers is like the difference between sex and masturbation. As the beard starts getting longer, the brush is indispensable in distributing the oil through the hair and getting oxygen to the surface of your face. This will keep your face from being either a pool of oil or a desert basin.

Wash your face with *extremely* mild soap. Again, a more thorough discussion of soap comes later in the book, but it's critical that you use mild soap so you don't dry your skin and hair out. Don't use shampoo with perfume. Don't condition yet. Don't use acne-medicated face wash. In fact, don't use your normal face wash at all. Get some handmade, natural soap from a farmer's market (Vegetable oil based, maybe five ingredients tops... Think hippie soap.). Put a hot washcloth on your itching beard to open up the pores of your skin below. Gently wash with a small lather of the soap. Finish with cold water on your face to close the pores back up. Keep your face moisturized: Use mild soap!

If after all these steps it's still itching, apply aloe vera gel to your face to soothe the itching and moisturize your skin. Aloe vera is natural and has countless benefits, especially for skin and hair. Some sources even claim that in some people, aloe vera can even assist hair growth. Aloe vera can only *help* your hair and skin, so you have nothing to worry about. I've found that mild, alcohol-free spray on toner can really help with keeping the itch at bay, as well.

Wait a week. The itching will pass, my son.

If you've followed these steps and your beard is driving you insane, try applying hydrocortisone or another medical-strength anti-itch cream. It's will be messy and disgusting, but you're going to be happy you didn't shave and become a disappointing failure for the rest of your life (And that's in your own eyes. Don't even get me started on what everybody else is going to think!). In extremely, and I mean, *extremely* rare situations, as in you're getting facial eczema or a horrible breakout, you might have to get rid of the hair or see a doctor. However, I'd still recommend growing it out past the itchy stage, because shaving is just going to make any skin condition worse: ten-fold.

All beards will itch when they come in. You know how a cut or scrape will itch as it heals? This your face healing.

Patches

Another complaint is that there are bald spots on your face where hair doesn't grow. Some men just don't grow facial hair in certain areas. It's up to you to decide what to do about it.

If the beard is mostly thick, let it come in and cover up the patchy parts by growing over them. A lot of men do not grow hair connecting their mustache with the rest of their facial hair, but it looks like their mustache is plenty long enough and must be rooted all the way to the beard.

Let the beard grow and just live with the patches. Once you've got enough of a beard, you can style it or sculpt it to avoid the patchy areas.

If it's still really patchy, wait to grow out facial hair later in life when your beard is thicker all over your face. No beard is better than a bad beard.

Grey Hair

Beards can age you or make you look younger, depending on how old you are, and what your beard looks like. A salt and pepper beard is generally considered to be very sexy and extremely stylish. Cinnamon and sugar (Red beard going grey) … Not so much.

Obviously, you can choose to embrace and live with your grey facial hair, but for a lot of men, a grey beard is going to add ten years, and that can be a real setback, image-wise.

If your beard is going grey for health reasons, get it together soldier! Passion's First Law: Healthy Man, Healthy Beard. Get healthy and eliminate stress. If it's genetic or natural for your age, don't worry. You have options.

Style your facial hair to avoid the grey patches. Going grey around your mouth? Sideburns it is. Grey neck beard? No more neck beard.

If you're only beginning to go grey, you can snip the grey hairs. Don't pluck them, as repeated plucking can lead to follicle death.

Most men choose to color their beard. There is an entire section in most drug stores for men's beard dyes, and if you select your color well, you can pull this off very easily. Just like a grey beard can add ten years to your look, a beard with full, uniform color *can take ten years off*. I highly recommend this for men in their 50's and 60's who want to look younger but have significantly grey beards. Facial hair dye must be made from the fountain of youth. My only caution is that you stay on top of your dyeing. Don't let your roots grow in so people see the grey hair growing in underneath, and don't pick a color that doesn't look right on you.

Negative Commentary

I hate to add to their negativity, but most people are pretty dumb. There is no better evidence to support this than what people say to you when you're growing a beard. There exists maybe five standard beard quips, and you're going to hear them from everyone (I'm not going to spoil the surprise, you'll hear them soon enough). Friends, coworkers, family, and even strangers all have something to say about it. By day two, you're going to be so bored of their banal attempts at wit that you're going to want to shave. You're obviously smarter than most people because you've broken out of their little box and you're trying something new. I also know you're smarter than most people because you're good at picking out books.

I've found that facial hair generally elicits positive response, so don't take a few negative cracks the wrong way. None of what people say is meant to be genuinely hurtful. The worst case is that they are jealous. Most of the time, people are just saying what they think people are supposed to say to someone growing out a beard. It's like those moments when someone's dressed up to go out on a date: *"Oooooh! Somebody's* got a date!" Some dumb-ass *always* has to make a cliché wisecrack. **In the beginning, your beard is going to be a dumb-ass magnet**.

The jealousy comes out because you're doing something awesome. Men who can't, or are afraid to, will chastise you in your efforts to grow facial hair because they are too weak to do it themselves. Beard envy is a serious issue, too. Psychologists and sociologists readily point out penis envy. Beard envy is almost the same thing, since the beard can symbolize many of the same masculine traits. Watch out for women with beard envy. They are rare, but they are fast with a blade.

A lot of time, people are afraid of what your beard may symbolize. You're not afraid to be an individual, to willingly accept the uniqueness of your face. You are an agent of social change and by it being on your face, it's now in their face. Most people can't handle even the slightest bit of change, and are painfully afraid to break from the easy monotony of conformity. You're making a commitment, *your own commitment*. I cannot praise you enough.

Most of the former facial hair stereotypes are crazy, scary characters. People might think you're one of those characters now, too. We can collectively quell this by taking care of our facial hair and dressing well and always presenting ourselves with poise and confidence. Your beard is going to look great because *you* look and feel great, and everyone in the room will know you're the man because of it. Awesome facial hair is just the icing on the being-the-man cake.

Here's how to handle negative commentary:

Consider the source. Ask yourself, "Who is this person and why are they saying this to me?"

Consider your beard. Does it suck? If it does, it's going to get better. Does it *really* suck? Do they have a point? See Passion's 4th Law.

Know why you're growing your beard. Even if you're just growing it for the hell of it, embrace that. You don't need to say much, but be ready to offer your defense. **Own the conversation: Be in command of it**.

Look presentable and be nice. If you're dressed well and you're a friendly guy, you'll have nothing to worry about. People are used to guys with beards being dirty and reclusive and weird. People have expectations going into anything, and since facial hair was effectively erased from mainstream culture, most people are going to expect the stereotypes when they talk to you. Smile and be nice first. When you're nice first, they're going to forget any beard stereotypes *instantly*, leaving you a fresh, friendly, and interesting person.

Women

Complications with women can arise in several ways. Problems can affect a current relationship, or the successful acquisition of new ones. Let's get the easy stuff out of the way first.

She Doesn't Like It

Tell her it's not finished yet. If you guys are close, she's going to be around while you grow out the beard, however long it takes to get the amount of growth you want. She's going to see it through the good and the bad.

Tell her it's the same as if she got a haircut you didn't like. That wouldn't change how you feel about her, so why should your beard change the way she feels about you? And just like the haircut will grow into something nice, so will your beard.

Whisker Burn

Your new whiskers can be harsh on your lover's face. Even women who are supportive to the cause can break down when they can't kiss their man without getting what feels like sandpaper to the face. Just like beard itch, this will go away soon.

Reassure her that this is only because the hair is so short. Once it's got some length, it gets *much* softer. Plus, being clean shaven will only make the whisker burn worse, as it will *always* be sprouting back out in its shortest, most rigid state. Also, she might want to up her facial moisturizer usage, which can prevent bad whisker burn, as well.

Appearance

You're only going to run into opposition if you don't take care of your beard. Keep your beard clean and keep it well groomed. The thought of smelly facial hair disgusts me, and will disgust any woman. Don't ever let your facial hair smell bed. EVER! Un-groomed facial hair will detract from your appearance, whereas well-groomed facial hair will make you look more put together than you might be. (Old school barbers are truly miracle workers in that sense: A good shave to clean up your style makes you look *damn good*).

Respect your lover by respecting yourself: Look good. Make her proud to be seen with you, and as proud of your face as you are.

Confidence

A lot of men mistakenly believe their facial hair is why women aren't interested in them.

We get this vicious cycle:

~~Boy~~ Man thinks woman won't like his beard,
Man loses confidence,
Women senses insecurity,
Women seeks out a more confident mate,
Man thinks woman didn't want him because of his beard.

As long as you don't look like a freak with it, most women don't care about facial hair. In fact, if you do it with style, you get bonus points. She'll only make an issue about it if you make an issue about it, first.

Women want confidence in their man. If you're a fun guy who has the balls to look the way he wants and can carry himself accordingly, you've got nothing to worry about. This is why women like musicians, it takes confidence to get up on a stage and pour your soul out.

It may be hard to look good and have confidence while you're in the early stages of growing out your beard, so you might have to wait until you've done with it what you want. On the other hand, you can use it to your advantage. Just like when you're traveling and you compare accents or languages, men and women love to discuss differences between the sexes. Comedians know it, screenwriters know it, matchmakers know it, and now you know it too. Let your new beard be a conversation starter. Ask a girl what she thinks about it. Get her talking. Everyone feels good when they're talking. Bam, you just made her feel good. Off to a great start!

Yes, there are women who are not going to like facial hair no matter what. Fine. There are plenty of fish in the sea, and you look like a fisherman now. Beards are awesome, right? So wouldn't it follow that a woman who agrees would be awesome too? Do yourself a favor and find a girl who will let you be yourself and love you for it.

A Warning

Your beard can never compensate for lack of character, it can only add to it. Be more than your beard. Have something to say in life. Your facial hair is just an accessory to your style, and a powerful form of self-expression. It's like a woman with huge boobs; yeah she's got awesome knockers, but there's probably a lot more to her than her boobs. There had better be more to you than your beard. What's behind your beard?

Life in the Pash Lane

My beard has been instrumental in helping me live up to the name "Passion."

Bad Beard Days

While beards grow in, they vacillate between looking great and looking not-so-great. Some areas will be thicker than others. Even while you're just growing out the beard, before you've done anything with it, you can have bad beard days. It doesn't matter what it is, some days it's not going to look as good as you know it can, for reasons outside of your control.

Humidity, wind, heat, rain, weird smells, and countless other unpredictable forces will work against you and your beard. However, if every day is a bad beard day, shave it off and start again later. Facial hair already has a bad reputation, and we've got to clean up the streets. This is mostly directed at younger beardsmiths: If you're not ready to grow a beard, use discretion, and wait until you can to do it right. It's critical that if you're going to do this, you do it well; for your sake, for all men's sake.

Key Points

- Itching is unavoidable, but it will pass and it's certainly manageable.

- Patchy beards can be managed, as well. However, if your beard is *really* patchy, you might just want to wait to grow a beard.

- Grey hair can add ten years to your age. Uniform color and stylish grooming can *take off* ten years. Facial hair dye is a great option for men with grey beards.

- Whisker burn goes away as facial hair gets longer and softer.

- Women won't care about your facial hair as long as it's well groomed and you're confident about it.

Part II: Grooming

Taste

There are thousands of ways you can style your facial hair, but first, you have to understand the basics.

Facial Hairstyles Overview

Until now, there has been little regulation in the naming and classification of facial hairstyles. Every slight variation has been given a name, and in most cases, multiple names. It's too confusing to remember them all and the silliness in naming only hurts our cause. Additionally, cultural differences preclude our ability to classify with the naming conventions most people have used so far. For instance, "Muttonchops" aren't "Muttonchops" outside America, and Americans don't grow "Imperial mustaches."

For the sake of clarity, let us agree there are only five basic types of facial hair. All facial hairstyles fall into one or more of these categories. Whatever you want to call it beyond that is up to you. Just don't go overboard with it. Most, but not all, people will understand what a handlebar mustache is, but you're just going to look like an idiot telling people your mustache is a "Dual whisking action soda sweeper." I would probably throw up on you if you said that to me. Sweep that up.

Clean Shaven
Entire face and neck is hairless and shaven at regular intervals to maintain hairlessness. Albeit super boring, this is the most common facial hairstyle.

Beard
A beard covers the entire face with facial hair extending from the hair line, over the cheeks, jaw line and chin. A beard usually includes a mustache, but it not a requirement. This is the only facial hairstyle that includes the hair grown on the neck, but more often than not, the neck is shaved.

Mustache
A mustache is any facial hair grown on the upper lip and optionally the side of the mouth, as long as it does not connect under the mouth. There are more variations of mustache than any other facial hairstyle. Some popular ones include the handlebar, the Dali, and the pencil.

Goatees or Partial Beards
A goatee is any hair grown on the chin. A goatee can include minimal growth on the cheeks, but it will not connect to the hairline or cover the entire cheeks and jaw line like a beard. Most goatees also grow around the mouth to connect to a mustache, encircling the mouth. These are called "Van Dykes." Soul patches, grown right under the bottom lip, are also considered goatees. If a goatee and mustache do not connect, they are considered independent entities: "He's got a sweet mustache and a long goatee." When connected, "goatee" will acceptably refer to the union of both: "He's got barbecue sauce in his goatee! He must be the one who ate the last of the ribs! Get him!"

Sideburns

Sideburns are two sections of hair on either side of the face, grown from the hairline down along the checks that do not continue to the chin or to the neck. Sideburns, even at their longest, should stop at the jaw line. They can connect to a mustache as long as the chin and neck are bare. When sideburns are very large, and cover most of the cheek, they're usually called muttonchops.

I encourage you to defy silly naming conventions and just call your facial hair by one of these five styles. By doing so, you eliminate the possibility of being lumped in with stereotypes associated with certain facial hairstyles, and you'll have a better chance of "owning" your style. Remember, facial hair is unique to its face, so even if you wear a mustache that looks like Zorro's mustache, you don't have to be Zorro.

Check out facialhairhandbook.com for updates and pictures of facial hairstyles.

Location, Location, Location

The five basic facial hairstyles all grow in different locations on the face, and picking a location has a profound effect on how facial hair will shape your face. Where and how long you grow your facial hair can radically alter your look, for better or for worse.

Facial hair lines will guide people's eyes where you want them. You can draw attention away from your nose, or to your mouth. Conceal and make up for undesirable facial features: You might have the roundest face with the most sagging double-chin ever, but groom yourself a sharp beard, and now you've got the best jaw line in the room.

The next page features a chart to help you in selecting which facial hairstyle will work best for you.

Facial Hairstyle Selection Based on Face

Facial Shape	Recommended Styles	Discouraged Styles
Round	Beard, Goatee, Sideburns A beard can square up a face, just as a goatee can define a round chin. Sideburns that don't flare too much can square up the face, too, and add length.	Beard A beard can also make the face too round. Keep it trimmed on the sides and get the length from the bottom and neck.
Square	Beard, Mustache A round beard or a round mustache (Think handlebar) will add the swooping round lines that can balance out an otherwise boxy face.	Sideburns, Goatee Sideburns tend to enforce square lines. You could get away with mutton chops with a round base though. Most goatees are just little boxes around the mouth and will make you look like a blockhead.
Short	Beard, Goatee Grow a beard that is longer on the bottom, and cover the chin with a goatee. This will add length to your face	Sideburns, Mustache Sideburns can highlight a small, undesirable chin, and a mustache can make your face look even shorter.
Long	Beard A full beard will round out the face for balance.	Sideburns, Goatee Sideburns narrow the face, and a goatee will add even more length, further narrowing and elongating the face.
Small	Goatee, Small Mustache Add length with a goatee, and size contrast with a slim mustache.	Sideburns, Beard Covering too much of it will make your face look even smaller.
Large	Sideburns, Beard, Large Mustache Sideburns and short beards will cover the large face without adding too much too it. Large mustaches can separate/break the face in half so it's not too much.	Goatee, Long Beard Facial hair that hangs off the face will just make your face and head look even bigger that it already does!

Length vs. Girth

Both are great, but girth wins every time. Anyone can grow a long beard, but robust facial hair takes care and attention. Thick facial hair is a sign of health and maturity. Facial hair gets thicker and thicker as you get older, and the only way to get healthy thick hair is to be healthy yourself. Of course, like everything, too much can be too much. Pick a style for your face, get it to a healthy length, and keep it there.

It takes a long time to grow long facial hair, and that means you're going to be wearing one style for a long time. Plus, hair naturally gets thinner at the ends due to breakage. That said, a long beard or goatee is an impressive symbol of long-term commitment; one that is authentic no matter what the trends are.

However, a long mustache, especially one that covers the upper lip, can be a nightmare. Things like eating and kissing can become exceedingly difficult, and the hairs constantly going in your mouth can drive you crazy. You're going to have to take extra care of a long mustache, and you'll likely want to style it daily.

Be careful not to get so focused on length that you end up having a bunch of thin hair. Biologically, hair thins when its host isn't healthy, so you're going to look sick if you've got straggly hair, even if you're in perfect health. A long nasty beard is going to make *you* look nasty; but a long healthy beard is going to stop traffic and inspire the world.

If you're going to go long, go strong.

The Three S's of Style

If you keep one simple rule in mind, you will have no trouble at all wearing your facial hair with style and confidence. If only fashion was this easy.

Passion's 4th Law of Facial Hair
Solid, Subtle, and Sharp

Solid

Having solid arrangements of hair is one of the easiest ways to make you and your facial hair look good. Keep your beard, sideburns, and goatees trimmed to avoid loose straggling hairs. Don't wear a style that will reveal bald patches.

Subtle

I advise against exotic facial hairstyles. While lightning bolt sideburns, initials carved into a beard, and multi-colored mustaches are fun, in normal day-to-day circumstances, they're just going to make you look like an idiot. We're trying to look stylish, and facial hair alone is exotic enough. Avoid extremes: Don't grow it too long or too bushy. Curl your mustache, but don't make complete circles. Think elegance, taste, and refinement. **You want your facial hair to give attention to your face, not take it all for itself**.

Sharp

Clean lines look clean and clean is king! Keep your beard sharp by keeping the lines well groomed. Whatever your facial hairstyle, shave or trim often to maintain your edges. Sharp lines completely dispel the myth that facial hair is for the lazy. In fact, keeping your facial hair sharp will actually make you look better because it highlights your attention to your appearance. Bonus.

Key Points

- There are five basic facial hairstyles. Everything is a variation or combination of those styles.

- Certain facial hairstyles work better than others for different faces.

- If you're going to wear it long, wear it strong.

- Passion's 4th Law: Keep your facial hair solid, subtle, and sharp.

- Don't use silly names for facial hairstyles.

Tools

Men love tools. Our caveman ancestors loved their bone axes and rock hammers, just like men today carry smartphones and work BBQs. Facial hair grooming is another excuse to stock up! And before you can begin grooming your facial hair effectively, you're going to need to assemble a toolkit. This chapter focuses on what you need and what it's for. You'll find the running theme is quality. I recommend you buy the best stuff you can afford, as it will not only do a better job, but in some cases, it will probably last you a lifetime.

Beard-wearers relax: Most of these tools involve shaving, but that's because unless you're going to wear a full beard, you're going to need to shave to maintain your facial hairstyle. For you, grooming is essentially the process of keeping your beard clean, and keeping it styled. A beard trimmer will be all you need to maintain your length and your neckline.

Wash Cloth

For washing your face and preparing your face for a shave, the washcloth is *indispensable*. You'll see why in the chapter entitled *Technique*. I'd recommend buying several white ones, because they're easy to wash in hot water, and so you'll always have a clean one.

Hand Towel

You're going to want a small towel set aside to dry your face off with after you wash and shave it.

Face Wash

For washing your face, you're going to need some face wash. Face wash usually has agents in it that help remove greasy oil from the face, which is great for making your face look clean, but will damage your facial hair. **We want to avoid face wash runoff at all costs**. If you're serious about facial skin care, you'll want to invest in a mild face wash for regular use, as well as an exfoliating scrub to use now and then. Facial skin care is an important part of looking good and staying young, and it's important here because of the extra scrutiny your newly-bearded face is receiving.

Electric Shaver

There are two ways to shave: A wet shave and a dry shave. A wet shave refers to preparing your face with shaving cream and using a razor blade to shave. A dry shave refers to using an electric shaver (sometimes mistakenly called an "electric razor," when there is no razor involved) and does not require any preparation. Both have their advantages and disadvantages. This chart should spell it out for you...

	Speed	Shave
Dry Shave	Winner	Loser
Wet Shave	Loser	Winner

You can't beat an electric shaver for convenience (We're talking 20 seconds to shave your entire face and neck), but you'll never get the high quality, lasting shave you get with a wet shave.

An electric shaver is nice to have around if you're running late in the morning, because **it's better to shave with an electric shaver and maintain clean lines than to not shave at all**. If you can't take the time to do a good wet shave, at least you're doing something. However, you will definitely have a 5 'o clock shadow by mid afternoon. Don't get me wrong, a high quality electric shaver can give you a great shave, but it's never going to match the benefits of a wet shave.

An electric shaver can be nice for quick touch-up jobs too. For instance, if you're about to get in bed with your lover, and she's very sensitive to whisker burn, the electric shaver can clean you up before she gets a headache or decides she's too tired.

If you have sensitive skin, though, you're probably going to want to avoid an electric shaver. They go dull and most people don't keep them clean; two sure ways to irritate your skin. Some people switch to dry shaving because they think it's going to irritate their face less. If you're doing a wet shave properly, you won't get any irritation at all.

Some recent advances in electric shaver technology have combined the skin preparing benefits of a wet shave with the convenience of a dry shave. Find an electric shaver that will allow you to use pre-shave oil or shaving cream if you want to. Some models will even squirt shaving cream out for you!

Pre-Shave Oil

For protecting your face from the razor, lubricating the shave, and preventing razor burn, pre-shave oil is truly a miracle worker. Pre-shave oil is a frequently overlooked, yet inexpensive and easy-to-use shaving tool that can really improve the quality of shave and prevent skin irritation. Some products even include camphor, to heat the face to open the pores even more.

Shaving Creams and Gels

Shaving cream is an interesting topic.

Most men are used to shaving cream or gel that you purchase in a drug store. It's often sold in an aerosol can and foams up when you squirt it out. Do not under any circumstance buy this kind of shaving cream. It's full of chemicals and alcohol, and comes out of the can really cold, guaranteed to irritate your face and prevent getting a clean, close shave.

Some seasoned shaving veterans will go so far as to claim that warm water is enough to get a good shave. You can use oils to lubricate your shave and get good results, too. You can also just use a very basic soap. The function of shaving cream is to lubricate the shave and hold the hairs up so the blade can easily cut them.

I think shaving cream is a critical part of the shaving process, and I recommend going the high quality route. High quality shaving creams are basically soap: All natural oils with glycerin to make lather. They're mixed in a hot mug or a bowl and applied with a brush made of natural animal hair. Most shaving creams do more harm than they do help, which is why, honestly– it's an optional step. On the other hand, real shaving cream –the good stuff – will do you *a lot* of good.

If you're going to buy something at a drug store, or want to go a simpler route, use shaving gel. Shaving gel can be heated also, and it generally contains fewer chemicals than aerosol can cream. High quality, natural gel is available too. One nice thing about shaving gel is that it is usually transparent enough that it lets you see what you're doing while you're shaving around hair on your face. I generally recommend shaving gel for travel when your normal shaving regimen might be excessive.

Shaving Brush

You're going to need a brush to mix and apply your shaving cream lather. They're commonly made of badger or boar bristles. The function of the brush is twofold. First, obviously, to mix and apply the lather, but these brushes also fulfill an important role in exfoliating the skin and lifting the hairs for easy shaving.

Ceramic Mug

You can use a bowl instead, but shaving cream just looks so awesome in a mug!

Razor

Nothing says pro shaving like a straight razor. If shaving becomes an interest and hobby for you, shaving with a straight razor can be a very rewarding experience. I highly recommend visiting a barber and getting a straight razor shave at some point in your life.

A straight razor in perfect condition will give you a better shave than anything. However, straight razors need to be sharpened, honed and stropped. Unless you are a barber, the likelihood of your straight razor being kept in perfect condition is slim. Additionally, there is a great deal of technique involved with wielding a straight razor, which is difficult when shaving your own face.

For these reasons, it's almost always better to use a high quality disposable razor. A good razor will *reliably* give you almost the quality of a perfect straight razor shave. Leave the straight razor for hobbyists and professional barbers. (It should be noted, however, that a straight razor is vastly less wasteful, and is highly recommended for men who are conscious about the footprint they're leaving on the environment).

Disposable razors vary in quality. From cheap plastic fixed-blades, to multiple blade razors with articulating heads that contour to your jaw, all the way to a high-end single blade razors in a handmade, balanced handles.

Single blade razor shaving is as close as you will get to a straight razor shave. While replacement razors are inexpensive and usually available, the handles are not, and supplies are most often sold in specialty shaving shops. Single blade shaving uses what is called a "Safety razor," or a "Dual edge" or "Double edge" razor, sometimes abbreviated "DE." These razors began the societal transition away from ubiquitous straight razor usage. Safety blade shaving is generally considered old-fashioned, but remains a top pick for shaving enthusiasts and has really made a comeback in recent years.

Multiple blade razors are based on the idea that the first blade lifts the hair up from your face and the subsequent blades cut it off. This is in all likelihood just a marketing gimmick. Warm water and/or shaving cream make the hair stand up and more elastic, which is what lets you get a close shave. Furthermore, the blades are close together and get clogged very easily. However, the advantage of most of these popular razors is that they have heads that move to fit the contour of your face. This means you can get by with weak technique and not cut yourself; safety razors take a little getting used to and cost more to get started with.

This is a practical guide, and hobbyists and enthusiasts are usually not as concerned with practicality as they are with perfection. While I recommend the safety razor method (In the long run it's cheaper *and* faster), I am completely sympathetic to the fact that you have more important things to think about than the many different razor options available to you. Every man's face is different and every man's needs are different. The shaving tips in the *Technique* section apply no matter what blade you decide to use. Whichever route you go, there are couple important things to consider:

Your Razor Must Be Kept Razor Sharp

Whatever blade you use, it's useless if it has begun to dull. A dull blade will prevent a close shave, cause you to use too much pressure, and cause skin irritation. They're disposable for a reason. Dirty, dull blades are the cause of almost all shaving irritations. A sharp, simple blade is always better than a dull fancy one.

You Get What You Pay For

Everything in shaving is preparation and cleanup work for the single act of this blade being slid along your face. Don't skimp at the most critical link in the chain; Use good stuff. Good razor blades have more consistent edges and they stay sharp longer. Change them often. If you end up with a style that involves shaving often, it's worth it to invest in good kit.

Aftershave Products

After you're done shaving, it can be useful to use some facial toner to seal pores and remove impurities. Alcohol-based toners work great, but the alcohol is going to sting and dry your skin out. A better bet is a natural, alcohol-free facial toner. It'll be much easier on the skin, so you can get its refreshing benefits more often. There are also specialty post-shave toners. Aftershave is a toner, and it makes you smell good too. Again, shoot for alcohol-free, and just like everything else, as few and as natural ingredients as you can find.

Beard & Mustache Trimmer

Think of an electric trimmer as just a really light duty version of what a barber uses to shave your head. Trimmers have different sized snap-on heads that let you mow your beard to a certain length, just like you would your lawn. If you require keeping your beard, sideburns, or goatee at a certain length, you're going to use your trimmer all the time. Electric trimmers are vastly faster to use than scissors, but need to be kept in good condition to be effective. If you go this route, get a high quality model with high power (You're picking up on the trend here). I have seen cheap ones just chew at the hair instead of trim it!

For beard wearers, this might be the only tool needed. Check out facialhairhandbook.com for some more trimmer insights.

Scissors

You're going to need a pair (or a few pair) of scissors in your facial hair toolbox. Scissors are perfect for trimming facial hair to a certain length, especially mustaches. They afford you the precision an electric trimmer will never have. However, it takes a long time to trim a beard with scissors, and it's hard to keep it even.

High quality scissors require very little maintenance, especially since we're only cutting facial hair. Buy from barber supply stores or specialty knife shops to get the best quality.

They're great for eliminating split ends, too.

Shampoo vs. Soap

Washing your beard is going to be really important to keeping the hair and your face underneath it clean and healthy.

Most people wash their hair with shampoo and their skin with soap. Shampoo is different than soap in that it's a detergent. It's not oil-based like soap, and it's composed of chemicals that make a big lather. Soap is affected by water hardness, and in hard water situations, will cause soap scum (This is why people have soap scum in their showers). In your hair, this means it won't rinse out well, leaving behind residue that will cause you to have rough, dry, ugly hair. Shampoo is unaffected by the hardness of water, so it will wash right out.

Unfortunately, shampoo is extremely hard on your hair. Most shampoo, even high quality shampoo, is full of synthetic chemicals and perfumes. Your body makes oil to encase and protect the hair. Shampoo strips this oil from your hair, exposing it to irreversible damage. Shampoo companies can then sell you conditioner to make up for the damage their shampoo does. Plus, **when used on your face, shampoo can and will cause skin irritation**.

True soap is very simple. It's made from natural oils, and the production process does not include any harsh chemicals. Soap is great for cleaning your hair because it won't strip away any of the protective oils your body creates, but will effectively clean away any debris. It's also going to clean your face underneath, *and* sooth your skin; all without irritation! There's still the issue of soap scum. If you use soap, **you just have to make sure you really wash it out**. Real soap is the better option, but if you can't use it because your water is too hard, then you're going to have to use shampoo.

Do not, under any circumstances, use body soap, body wash, or deodorant soap on your face. Your facial skin can't take the abrasiveness, and the hair will dry out in no time. The fewer the ingredients, the better!

If you use shampoo, use high quality shampoo to minimize hair damage and facial irritation. Just like anything we've discussed, you get what you pay for with shampoos, too. High end, salon brands have simpler, more natural ingredients. I recommend you get some fresh, natural soap from a farmer's market or natural foods store and try it out. If the condition of your hair is getting rough, simply switch to shampoo.

Life in the Pash Lane

I've tried everything on my beard. Shampoos, conditioners, treatments... Everything. Switching to some natural hippie soap I got at a farmer's market to wash my beard was the single best thing I've ever done for it.

Conditioner

Conditioner definitely has a use for our hair, but you don't need to buy into the marketing hype. Conditioner came along when shampoo was invented. These "care" products weren't around for thousands of years and we still had great hair (See Passion's First Law). Conditioner is definitely optional, but you may find it useful for one thing.

Passion's 5ᵗʰ Law of Facial Hair
Hair Care is a Defensive Game

Remember: **Hair is dead**. No conditioner is going to make your hair *better*, but it can help prevent it from getting worse.

All we can do in caring for our facial hair, or any hair, is to prevent it from getting worse. One way to make it worse is to let stuff get in it. In the shower, and especially when you use shampoo, the scales of your hairs become very porous and open. Conditioner flattens those scales down, like closing the pores of your face, preventing particles of stuff from getting into your hair and damaging it.

Good conditioner can be instrumental in keeping your dead hair looking as good as it did the day it came out of your face. Cheap stuff, on the other hand, will actually go into the hair and ruin it. What makes good conditioner? Quality, simple ingredients. Oil alone will decrease the porosity of your hair, and can be used as a fantastic conditioner, but commercial conditioners are much easier to use, especially in a shower. Try the beauty isle of your natural foods store, again. "Beard-specific" products, while available, are unfortunately no different than normal products.

Treatments

There are whole aisles in stores stocked with hair treatments. You can experiment with as many of them as you like, but most of them will damage your hair.

I generally advise against treating your hair at all, just grow healthy hair and keep it clean and trimmed. Moreover, most of you won't have *that* much hair on your face, so don't worry about it. When your hair starts to get long, a hot oil treatment can act as a really serious conditioning. The metaphor I like to use is like using sealant on a wooden deck. Your deck may be damaged from the elements, but applying some sealant will at least prevent it from getting any worse.

Any oil will work. Jojoba oil is generally considered to be the "hair oil." Some people like to use olive oil, still others sesame. Some people swear by mayonnaise or even peanut butter! I've had the best experiences with and recommend jojoba oil for hair, but you might prefer others. I'll discuss how to treat your hair with jojoba oil in the *Technique* section.

Facial Moisturizer

The top layer of your skin is actually all dead skin, so while being hydrated definitely helps, you can still get dry skin. Research has shown that facial moisturizers keep your skin elastic and supple, which keeps you wrinkle free and looking young. Good technique will prevent it as much as possible, but shaving can dry your skin out, so after you apply toner or aftershave, put on some face lotion. Keeping your skin moisturized is also a great way to prevent razor burn or other skin irritations caused while shaving.

A lot of facial moisturizers also include sunscreen. No matter your skin color, you are susceptible to sun damage on your skin. Sun damage is the leading cause of a lot of skin issues, most notably premature aging. Select an SPF rating high enough for your skin color, and wear facial lotion with sunscreen daily to ensure healthy glowing skin that will stay with you for years to come.

You don't need to put lotion on the parts of your face that are covered by facial hair.

Brushes

A hairbrush is a simple tool. As stated earlier, its function it to stimulate your scalp and move the oil found at the scalp throughout the hair.

Any high quality boar-bristle hairbrush will suffice for what you're going to be using it for. Avoid plastic brushes as they will pull your hair to the point of snapping, charge it with static electricity, and catch and pull your hair out at the root.

Combs

If you've got some length to your facial hair, you're going to need a comb to detangle it. Also, if you're using scissors to trim, a comb is great to use to cut against.

Avoid plastic combs, as they will snag your hair just like a plastic brush. Instead opt for a readily available Bakelite comb. Some people prefer materials like bone or wood, but Bakelite combs are inexpensive, readily available, and are guaranteed to be seamless.

You might want to have a couple of different sizes. Small, fine-toothed combs are great for styling a mustache, but might snag in a thick beard.

Styling Aids
Mustache Wax

Good mustache wax is basically really strong, waxy pomade. It's actually not too bad on your hair, especially considering how well it gets your mustache out of your mouth. Good mustache wax doesn't even cost that much. Avoid chemicals and dyes and you should be set. Facialhairhandbook.com has great recommendations and reviews of different mustache waxes.

Hairspray

Some people will argue that the alcohol in hairspray will not get on the hair because it evaporates in the spray, and that the ingredients in hairspray will actually protect your hair. Some people will also argue that the world is flat. Hairspray will hold your facial hair the way you want it, but not without the cost of drying out your hair. The process of washing it out is also damaging.

Gel and Mousse

Gel has all of the drawbacks of hairspray and none of the benefits. Besides, it's too heavy to use in facial hair. Mousse will add texture, but it's really just not for facial hair. No need for either.

Pomade

Pomade will work just like wax, and unless you need to hold your mustache very tightly, is a great way to have a more natural look while still holding the hair into a style.

Other

Men's shaving is full of interesting products. Just like our simplified discussion of facial hairstyles, so is our discussion of tools. These tools will help you groom facial hair very practically, but if something catches your eye, try it out. Tools are fun, and shaving tools are often the first tools we get to play with every day. Different brands of razors have different characteristics, just like different shaving brushes can work better on different kinds of skin. You're going to have to try them out to decide what works best for you.

Don't worry if you can't put together an amazing facial hair toolbox right away. This is stuff you will collect eventually, and like I said, probably keep forever.

Key Points

- Buy high quality products and focus on natural, simple ingredients.

- Wet shaving and dry shaving both have their merits, but wet shaving wins for a close shave.

- It's better to shave with an electric shaver and maintain clean lines than to not shave at all.

- Invest in a safety razor for great shaves.

- Experiment with different products and brands to find what works best for you. Everyone's different.

- Passion's 5th Law: Hair Care is a Defensive Game. Play some strong D, homey.

Technique

This chapter highlights the basic grooming techniques used in styling and maintaining good facial hair.

Some men spend an entire lifetime honing these techniques. Keep things simple and strive for consistency, not perfection. Don't get too wrapped up in the details if doing so is going to prevent you from doing anything!

Cleaning and Care

Washing Your Exposed Face

Washing and shaving are almost the exact same things except you don't use your razor when you wash your face.

1. Wash your hands.
2. Soak a washcloth in warm water. Don't use water that's too hot or you can damage your skin.
3. Apply the warm washcloth to face to open pores. Repeat until face feels noticeably warm and soft.

Follow your face wash's instructions on how much to use. Rub the cleanser in your hands until it lathers. Lightly scrub your face for 15-30 seconds.

4. Gently wipe cleanser off with washcloth. Wiping ensures you will remove the debris you cleaned off. **It also prevents facial cleanser from washing into your facial hair.** This is important!

5. Soak the washcloth in cool water and apply to face to close pores.

6. Optionally follow up with alcohol-free toner.

7. Moisturize your exposed face with facial moisturizer.

Washing Your Hair

1. Wet hair with warm water. Don't use water that's too hot or you can damage the hair or the face.
2. Lather soap in hands, or squirt out some shampoo.
3. Work soap/shampoo all through hair with fingers, making sure to massage the face.
4. Wash soap/shampoo out completely with cold water. This will help to close the cuticle of the hair, and the pores of the face underneath it.
5. Let the hair air dry while you continue to do other things. For longer facial hair, pat dry.

Conditioning

1. If you have just washed your hair with warm water or shampoo, apply conditioner.
2. Work conditioner throughout hair.
3. Let it sit on the hair while you wash something else.
4. Rinse the conditioner out with lukewarm or cold water.

Treating (For Longer Facial Hairstyles)

1. Heat 1 Tablespoon of jojoba oil. Putting some in a hot cup or heating a cup of oil in a sink of hot water... Whatever works... Just don't microwave it!
2. Coat the hair with the warm jojoba oil. Massage it into the hair and face.

3. If possible, wrap the beard in a plastic shower cap. Let the oil sit on the hair for 3-5 minutes.
4. Wash the oil out with the hair washing steps above. Optionally, you can just rinse the oil out with cool water, but it will be very oily afterward, and not to worry, the washing won't undo the effects of the treatment.

Combing
Combing your facial hair is really only necessary if it gets long.
1. Wait for hair to dry. Never comb or brush wet hair, as it is extremely elastic and will snap.
2. Start at the bottom of the hair and comb outward to remove tangles and snags. Move up each time working your way to the face.

Brushing
1. Wait for hair to be dry. If you have a long beard or goatee, **never brush wet hair!** Wet hair is super elastic and will stretch and snap.
2. Start at the face and brush outwards to distribute oil throughout hair. Use long strokes. If you have a long beard or goatee, you will need to detangle it first with a comb.
3. Don't over-brush; you'll damage the hair. Once or twice through, all over the face, should be enough.

Protection
If you're going swimming, or are going to spend a lot of the day in the wind or sun, you can protect your facial hair by putting lightweight oil in it. Shea butter is also *fantastic* for protecting your hair, and even has some sun protection ability. If you've grown good hair and are taking good care of it, you should be fine; beards are like human weatherproofing.

If you've got a long beard or goatee, braiding it is also a great way to keep it protected and out of the way.

Shaving

Shaving around your facial hair will keep you looking sharp. Wet shaving is essentially a three part procedure, which is very similar to washing your face:

Pre-Shave

1. Wash face as normal, but don't rinse with cool water yet.
2. Prepare your shaving cream in your mug.
3. Soak a washcloth in warm water.
4. Apply warm washcloth to face to open pores.
5. Apply a thin layer of pre-shave oil to the areas you want to shave.
6. Apply the warm washcloth again. If it's cooled, reheat it. You want to keep those pores open!
7. Apply shaving cream to your face. Use circular motions as well as dabbing. The shaving cream should be warm and the lather should be really foamy.

Shave

1. If using a safety razor, apply the safety bar (part of the handle), and then apply the blade at about a 30° angle against your face. For other razors, apply the head of the razor to your face.
2. Do not apply any pressure whatsoever! Let the weight of the handle drag the blade against your face. Applying pressure is the number one cause for shaving error.
3. For thin hair, use long strokes. For thick hair, use short strokes.
4. Between strokes, rinse the blade off in the sink, a bowl of water, or under running water.
5. Shave flat surfaces. It may help to conceptualize your face into separate regions for this. It also helps to stretch your face out with your non-razor hand. This stretching technique will be almost a requirement for your neck.
6. Ask yourself if it's worth all the work when you could grow an awesome beard.
7. For experienced shavers with really thick hair, re-lather and shave across or against the grain. I don't

recommend this for most guys, as it usually results in skin irritation.

Post-Shave

1. Rinse entire face with cool water to close pores.
2. Optionally, use a toner or astringent to seal pores and remove impurities. Quality aftershave will accomplish this and make you smell good at the same time.
3. Apply a facial moisturizer.

Shaping and Sculpting

My best advice for carving your beard into a style is to see a reputable barber initially. The barber will be able to sculpt the lines in the hair with the precision of an objective eye. Also, they're going to give you a really clean shave, which is a great start, easy for you to maintain afterward!

If you do it on your own, try these steps:

1. Decide what you want by drawing on pictures of yourself with no beard, or by using image editing software on a computer. Refer to the chart on style selection in the *Location, Location, Location* section of *Taste* for recommendations on what will work with your face. Don't be afraid to break those rules, though.
2. Draw "lines" in your beard hair with a comb. By now, you should have enough beard hair that you can separate it with the comb. Go for symmetry by using landmarks on your face. For instance, "I want my sideburns to line up with my nose," or "My beard is going to stop above my Adam's apple." Unless you're a mutant shape-shifter and your face radically changes, these kinds of measurements are easy to maintain later on.
3. Use your trimmer with no spacer to give yourself a rough shave along those guidelines. This is like using some clippers to give someone a buzz haircut. This will remove the bulk of the hair allowing for an easy shave.
4. Shave the remaining stubble off.

Trimming

- Snip split ends as they come.

- You don't have to trim every time you shave, but you need to make it a regular thing. See the Timing section for recommendations as to when to trim your facial hair.

- Always trim less off than you think you need to. It always grows back, but it's easier to just not mess up in the first place.

- Plucking hairs out can eventually kill the follicle, preventing any hair growth from that point from occurring ever again. It takes a few times for this to happen, but you should avoid plucking anyway.

- Remember Passion's 4th Law: Solid, Subtle, and Sharp. Keep your style solid by using your electric trimmer, and keep it sharp by shaving around it.

Key Points

- Washing is as easy as 1-2-3.
    1. Open pores
    2. Wash
    3. Close pores

- Shaving is as easy as 1-2-3.
    1. Pre-shave
    2. Shave
    3. Post-shave

- See a professional barber for your initial styling!

Timing

Make it a regimen, a routine, and most importantly, a ritual.

Shaving

Shave as often as you need to. Most men will want to shave every morning to keep things sharp and stylish. Looking good requires upkeep. You can shave twice a day if you need, but if you're going to do so, it's critical that you follow all the steps of a wet shave to avoid irritation. Shave in the morning so you look good all day.

Replace Razor Blades

Until you can begin to tell that your blade is going dull, you should replace your blade weekly. For cheaper razors, you might need to replace after one or two uses. Set aside some man time one day a week to take care of a few things.

Trimming

Trim your facial hair weekly, maybe when you replace your razor blade. Giving yourself a week will give your hair enough time to grow out so that you can really see what needs the trimming and what doesn't.

Washing

If you're using shampoo, don't wash too often. Soap (Again, not your usual body soap), as long as you rinse it out well, should be fine for light, daily washing. You can definitely over-wash and damage your hair with shampoo, but this is hard to do with weak soap. You can go a few days without washing and it won't hurt your hair one bit but I caution against this because your facial hair is likely to be under close scrutiny. **Don't even let people see it dirty even once or they'll think it's always dirty**.

Exfoliate your exposed face with a facial scrub or a mask once a week.

Conditioning

You should condition any time you use shampoo, and ideally anytime you get your beard wet with hot water. Washing your face and your facial hair, as well as shaving, always finishes with closing pores. The same should hold for your hair's cuticle.

Treatment

Treat your facial hair weekly to keep it clean and soft. Remember Passion's 5th Law: Hair Care is a Defensive Game. Think of a jojoba oil treatment as a really nice conditioning. Even once a month is going to make a difference in your hair's ability to protect itself.

Change it Up

If you find a style you really like, wear it as long as you want. This is how facial hair becomes iconic. If you like to experiment with new styles, or just keep things fresh, start the process over every three months. That'll give you a month to get your beard going, and two months to wear your style.

Key Points

- Take time every week to trim, change razor blades, and treat your hair. Make it a regimen, a routine, and a ritual.

- Don't over-wash your facial hair.

When Things Get Hairy

Ingrown Hairs

If you're following my advice to a tee, and you still get ingrown hairs, get a pair of needle-nose tweezers and pull the ingrown hair out. Keep your face and beard washed, and stop shaving until the ingrown hair heals. Ingrown hairs happen when you shave with a dull or dirty blade, or have really curly facial hair. Black men can get ingrown facial hairs very easily. Ingrown hairs usually start in the beginning of beard growth, so brush regularly to stimulate the face, manage oil, and keep the hairs from embedding themselves in your face.

Acne

A healthy diet and proper face washing technique are your best steps to prevent acne. If you're breaking out, drink a lot of water, and brush the beard to move the oil throughout. Stop shaving until the acne is under control. When you do shave, definitely use an astringent or toner afterward. And abide Passion's First Law, dude.

Beard Rash

Follow the proper wet shaving technique and you won't have to worry about beard rash. If you use a dirty, dull blade, apply too much pressure, and don't keep your face clean, you deserve all the beard rash you can give yourself. Soothe beard rash by washing the area with mild soap. Use an astringent or toner to prevent further infection. You can apply antibiotic ointment if it's bad, as well. Stop shaving until it heals, then use a new blade and follow the proper technique.

Nicks

Wet and apply a styptic pen or alum block to your wound. It will sting a little, but the bleeding will stop and the wound will hopefully close and not get infected. Stop using so much pressure with your razor!

Dry Skin

You usually get dry skin by over-washing, or by failing to moisturize after you shave. This is another reason I recommend soap instead of shampoo. Your facial skin is the most sensitive skin on your body after your genitals. Clean lightly!

If you're starting to flake and it looks like you've dandruff in your beard, supplement your diet with flaxseed oil and fish oil.

Good hydration will prevent dry skin from occurring, but the top layer of skin is just a bunch of dead skin cells. Exfoliate to remove the dead cells, and then moisturize. Avoid processed sugar and get enough sleep, too.

Itching

Still having problems with your beard itching? Make sure you're eating right, add the flaxseed oil and fish oil supplements, and brush three times a day. Itching that takes place after the beard has already grown out past its initial itchy stage is the result of a skin condition trying to heal itself, including but not limited to dry skin. Treat it the same way. Make sure you're washing your face underneath when you're washing your facial hair. Don't blow dry and avoid hot water!

Split Ends

Split ends are a problem because they look bad and they snag when you're combing or brushing, thus ripping the entire hair out of its follicle. Do that enough and your hair will give up trying to grow in that hole! Left un-trimmed, split ends will continue to break all the way back to the root of the hair.

Prevent split ends by growing good hair to begin with and by using good products on your hair. Fix split ends with your scissors as soon as you see them, or make it part of your regularly scheduled facial hair maintenance.

You Cut Off Too Much

Don't worry! It always grows back! Did you just trim it too close? Did you ruin the symmetry of your style? I hate to say it, but you might have to start over, or at least trim things way back. Maybe you can salvage what's left into a different style? In the future, prevent this by using an electric trimmer, and by holding the hair up with a fine-toothed comb. Measure what you want to cut or trim by landmarks on your face.

Keep up with your clean shaving lines so that you don't have to redefine your edges. More men cut off too much just trying to get back to what they had before they got lazy, than do when initially carving their style.

Boredom

Are you getting bored of your style? Shave it! One of the best things about facial hair is that it's temporary. Grow out another style. Try something different.

If you're growing your facial hair for a cause or in a contest, and you want to shave it, read the first chapter of this book, and consider how awesome what you're doing is. Awesome is as awesome does, amigo.

Eating and Drinking

Always take a couple extra napkins. Be conscious of the bite you're taking and where the fork is aiming. Open your mouth wide. Every man gets some food in his facial hair sometimes. Keep your mustache groomed and your beard tame and you can minimize the probability of food not making it into your mouth. Use a napkin after every bite if you have to.

Have a long mustache? Order drinks with a straw so you don't pour the drink on your mustache every time you take a swig. I can keep my mustache styled through the greasiest burger, but as soon as I get water on that mustache wax, it's a lost cause.

If you get food (or heaven forbid milk or ice cream) in your beard or mustache, go to the bathroom and wash it out. You don't want that smell so close to your nose.

Eating and drinking gets much easier as you get used to wearing facial hair. Practice makes perfect, so practice with healthy foods.

Elements

Wind

Wind can just *ravage* a beard or long goatee. Tie it up, use bobby pins to clip it to your face, do whatever you have to do to prevent it from getting whipped around in the wind. Wind will blow debris into your facial hair, and if it's long enough to be whipped around, wind give you split ends. Before you go in the wind, work some oil or shea butter onto the hair.

Sun
The sun will naturally highlight your hair, and it looks great. Again, it's essential that you grow out good hair to begin with, because it's not like we can just put sunscreen on our beard. The sun can dry hair out, just like it can to skin. Just moderate your sun and you can avoid dry hair. The hair will protect itself as best it can; learn to embrace the highlights. Try some shea butter on the tips for extra protection.

Rain
Rain is an issue for mustache men because it is the natural enemy of mustache wax. Bring an umbrella with you when it rains or move somewhere dry.

Humidity
Your facial hair will frizz out and open its cuticle in hot, damp conditions. Conditioner can really help undo these effects.

Chlorine
If you go swimming or sit in a hot tub, you're going to get a lot of chlorine on your facial hair. If you've got good healthy hair that you take care of, you won't have an issue. Make sure you wash the chlorine off afterward with mild soap and you'll be fine. A hot tub can damage hair just because the water's so hot, but it's usually only an issue with extremely long beards and goatees that sit in the water.

Dry Hair
If your hair is dry and crinkly and feels more like tinder than it does hair, you need to do a jojoba oil treatment as soon as possible. Then eat well, stimulate your face, and brush your natural oil throughout the hair. Dry hair is hard to fix. Don't over-wash or over-brush.

It's Too Hot Under All This Facial Hair

If you can't handle the heat, get out of the kitchen. A beard might make you a little warmer in the summer months, but it's nothing a man can't handle biologically.

Beard Gets Caught in Something

Assuming you've got a long enough beard for it to get caught in something, grab the beard above where it has been grabbed and hold as tight as you can. Pull and let the bottom of your beard get ripped off and sucked into the machine or fan or whatever it is that's got you. This is going to happen in a split second. You're going to lose a fat chunk of beard, but that's a lot better than your entire beard *and* a fat chunk of your face.

Beard Catches On Fire

Do not stop, drop, and roll like you've been told. If you do, you'll burn your face, too. Douse your face in water immediately. Don't use alcohol or you will burn your face! Hopefully someone will get a picture, because **you're going to look pretty hardcore!**

Afterward, you're going to need to trim off a lot of the hair, because it's going to smell bad, melt together, and break. It always grows back.

Lice, Ticks, and Fleas

I have never heard of anyone having an issue with fleas, ticks, or lice with facial hair, but you basically have two options: Shave it off and start over, or use the killer shampoos. I say go for the shampoo first. Those shampoos can be very damaging to the hair and more importantly the skin underneath, but it may work and then you'll be glad you didn't shave.

Terminal Beard

Facial hair, like all hair, will only grow so long. A lot of times, men's hair starts to break off at a certain point, but if you've been healthy for the duration of your beard growth, and your beard won't grow any longer, you've probably reached terminal beard. Terminal beard happens at different lengths for different people, and it's completely natural. Nothing is wrong with you; it's just your genes. You should never allow yourself to get to terminal beard, though, because you want to keep your beard solid. The hairs will stop growing at different lengths, and that's going to look scraggly and unkempt. You're almost at the end of this book, you should know better than that by now!

Going Grey

If you're going grey prematurely and are unhappy about it, go buy a facial hair dye kit and solve the problem.

It could also be the result of a nutritional deficiency. For instance, red-bearded men need enough beta carotene to ensure that they can grow the hair red. If you're taking a multivitamin, you're going to get everything you need. Passion's First Law prevents most of these complications. If you suspect something else is going on, see a doctor.

Thinning

Hair thinning is a sign that something's not healthy. It can be a nutritional deficiency (commonly protein or zinc in this case), or something more serious. Stress will also cause your facial hair to start thinning. If you suspect something else is going on, see a doctor.

Harassment

Look good and dress well and nobody will call you a terrorist, I promise. Smile first and be friendly. Cut through the stereotypes with the precision of your straight razor by being a stylish, confident man. Remember, nobody is genuinely trying to be mean; they're usually just too dumb to think for themselves and are just saying what they think people are supposed to say.

Post Traumatic Shaving Disorder

PTSD is a serious deal. If you are having nightmares, and wake up stroking the air below your chin, seek out community at facialhairhandbook.com. Care is there.

Afterword

This book is just the beginning. Most of the concepts and tips presented here are commonly known and generally accepted; some are the result of my own experience. There is a lot more to learn about diet, exercise, dating, and even shaving. I hope you will take every opportunity to make yourself a better man.

There have been a few themes in this book that I'd like to highlight in conclusion:

Good health is vital, whether or not you ending up wearing facial hair. It is paramount to confidence and success, and like most things, is a lot easier than you may think.

Facial hair is just an element of your personal style. *How* you wear your facial hair and your clothing is more important than what facial hairstyle you pick, or what clothes you wear.

Simplicity is also extremely important. Choose consistency over perfection, and don't make things harder than they need to be. Your facial hair is a simple and natural thing, which will serve to remind you that simple and natural are almost always the right choice.

Facial hair is a big part of what makes you a man and the growth of which is a valuable life experience. And I hope you will agree: Growing a beard is growing a man.

Appendix A:
Passion's Beard

I was four years old the first time I shaved. My father has had a mustache my entire life, and I would watch him shave his cheeks and neck in the mornings and the evenings before going out. One summer afternoon, I felt I was ready to be a man, so I went into the bathroom, took his razor, and went for it. Don't get me wrong, I was an expert with the shaving cream, but I had neither facial hair nor experience with a razor, so I ended up slitting my upper lip! Blood poured out and I screamed! Fortunately, it didn't scar physically, but maybe it left a deeper scar...

I really started growing facial hair at age twelve. I'm not an extremely hairy man – nor has anyone been in my ancestry – I just grow a lot of red facial hair, really fast. Like most boys, I started with shaving cream, a Bic® razor, and a father telling me what I was doing wrong. I later moved to an electric razor, returned to a real razor, and then quit razors cold turkey.

I began my facial hairstyles with sideburns. I was a fan of the '70s detective look: Polyester, western shirts, twill pants, aviator sunglasses, with long hair parted on the side, and big, big sideburns (I was young, I was wild. I had no style.). I could never grow much of a mustache, but during my sophomore year of high school, I grew out my first beard. It didn't get long, because I kept it short with a beard trimmer. Like most young men, I gave in to social and maternal pressures and shaved it off. I would re-grow and then continue to rock big sideburns until the end of my freshman year of college.

Bored of the mutton chops, I shaved them off and grew out another beard in early May of 2003, with the complete intention of harvesting it into a different style. I ended up shaving off that beard, and really regretting it. So at the end of that May, I started another beard, promising myself not to shave until it really grew in.

I had a very relaxing summer. I played music every day, and hung out in the beautiful California sun. I had a supportive girlfriend, no job or summer school for the first time in years, and life was easy. My beard grew out huge. When I came back in the fall, it was like I was a returning hero. Everyone loved my thick red beard! It would have been a social tragedy if I shaved, so I just kept growing my beard. It just kept getting longer and thicker and more red and beautiful. It was at this time that a friend of mine and I heard about the 2003 World Beard and Mustache Championships. It was being held in Carson City, NV, only a five-hour drive from my university. I decided not to go at the last minute. After the competition, there were pictures on the Internet, and I immediately regretted not attending. I would have done very well in a smaller-beard category, but more importantly, I would have had a great time. I vowed to go to the next World Beard and Mustache Championships no matter what.

Two years later, I found myself in Berlin at the 2005 World Beard and Mustache Championships. I won 3rd place in the Natural Full Beard division. It was quite an upset when some cowboy American kid, dressed in a last-minute Halloween pirate costume took such high honors in the most prestigious category in the contest. Beard Team USA captain, and my coach, Phil Olsen would later tell me that the Germans thought I was completely un-serious and disrespectful: It was the most patriotic thing I had done in my entire life.

Germany was a turning point for me in a couple of ways. One, I was now very conscious of facial hair, on myself and on others. My beard had always just been my beard, now it was something that I thought and talked about with people. Two, I was now, whether I liked it or not, an important face in the world of facial hair (Puns always intended).

Two years would pass before the next world championships. In that time, I had numerous television appearances and competed all over the country in beard competitions. As my beard grew longer, so did my list of titles. Beard competitions were my game, and I was on top of my game. This newfound attention to my beard led me to take better care of it. I learned a lot, mostly through trial and error, about what made my beard grow, for better or worse, and what I could do to take care of it.

Every one of my beard hairs is an antenna to the bearded world. I know who's out there and what they've got on their face. So I knew going into the 2007 world championships that it would be me against one other guy for first place. He had a much, much longer beard, but it was thin and grey. I've done well because of the intense thickness and red color of my beard. Being half the age of the next youngest competitor has probably helped too. I remember going to pre-judging, where they check to make sure you're in the right category, and seeing him there surrounded by cameras already. I returned to my hotel room disheartened, to dress and get ready for what I thought was going to be an epic failure. When I walked back and into the arena for the competition, I remember feeling this incredible negative vibe. Friends I had made on the trip, and even some of the Europeans I befriended in Germany, *wouldn't even look at me!* These people were taking it way too seriously. I was so turned off by the whole thing, I was almost sick. I sat down in the audience to avoid the chaos, but the chaos came to me...

I wore a brilliant white tuxedo. Accented with baby blue accessories, I had quite the costume. People loved it! I must have taken 5,000 photos with people that day. There was literally a line of people waiting to talk to me. Being surrounded by happiness and bombarded with admiration made me forget about the negative competitive vibes in the room. When I went up on stage to compete, I was having the best day of my life and I was confident no matter the outcome. The outcome, however, was that I won first place in the natural full beard category! Americans took first place in four other categories. It was a great success.

After Brighton, I started the research needed to augment my own experience for what would become the book you're reading right now.

In 2009, I won first place natural full beard again, and 3rd overall at the World Championship in Anchorage, Alaska. Americans like the underdog, so it was hard going into the competition a champion, but obviously not hard enough.

You get your hair genes from your maternal grandfather. My mom always told me her dad wore a big, bright red handlebar mustache. Thus, maybe facial hair was my destiny before I was even born. Have I fulfilled my destiny, though? I've had a lot of success with my facial hair, even if it's just because it has been so essential to my personal style and image; there's no way around it, for a musician, image is at least half the game. I've traveled the world, been all over TV, and people know who I am wherever I go. I get a lot of attention, but c'mon, it's a beard: It keeps me humble. I've made friends everywhere I've gone and made a pretty good life for myself. Growing a beard has been the best thing I've ever done...

...But I *am* open to shaving. It's a decision I could never make on my own so look for Jack Passion's Shave-It-Or-Save-It charity extravaganza one day in the future. I hope you've enjoyed this book, and I'd love to hear from you, so check out my music at jackpassion.com and keep updated on facialhairhandbook.com. Until then, take care...of your face.

Love,
Passion

Life in the Pash Lane
Finding that "Piratenkostume" (German for "Pirate Costume") was an adventure that took me, my friends, and a cameraman all over Berlin, and ended up with us running from the polizei. I'll leave you to guess what "Polizei" translates to.

Appendix B:
Passion's Laws of Facial Hair

1. Healthy Man, Healthy Beard

2. Good Facial Hair Starts With a Beard

3. Hair Growth is About Potential

4. Solid, Subtle, Sharp

5. Hair Care is a Defensive Game

About the Author

Jack Passion is the two-time world champion of beards. He won the title at the World Beard and Moustache Championships in Brighton England in 2007 and again in Anchorage, Alaska in 2009. Passion and his beard have been on The Tonight Show with Jay Leno, Good Morning America, The View, Regis and Kelly, and countless news segments, at home and abroad. Magazines as varied as TIME and Vice have had his facial fur grace their pages, and he has been profiled in every major newspaper. Passion is considered one of the world's leading experts on facial hair.

Jack holds a degree in Philosophy from the University of California at Santa Cruz. He lives in the San Francisco bay area where he is a musician, a writer, and an entrepreneur. *The Facial Hair Handbook* is his first book.

Learn more at facialhairhandbook.com and jackpassion.com.

Made in the USA
Lexington, KY
22 November 2013